Real Health

THE ILL EFFECTS OF STRESS AND THEIR PREVENTION

*

Real Health

*

THE ILL EFFECTS OF STRESS

AND THEIR PREVENTION

*

Dr Alex Poteliakhoff

AND

Dr Malcolm Carruthers

Davis-Poynter *London*

First published in 1981 by
Davis-Poynter Limited
20 Garrick Street London WC2E 9BJ

ISBN 0 7067 0246 8

Printed in Great Britain by Bristol Typesetting Co Ltd,
Barton Manor, St Philips, Bristol

Contents

*

We would like to record our grateful thanks to the late Heinz Nordin, who read the manuscript with an expert eye and made some valuable suggestions, to Mark Arnold Forster, who deleted obscure scientific language unfit for the intelligent layman, to Dr Fotherby of the Department of Steroid Biochemistry, Hammersmith Hospital, who very kindly carried out the cortisol estimations and to Diana, who did most of the typing.

Introduction

*

MODERN SCIENTIFIC MEDICINE, which has rapidly evolved over the past century has, without doubt, brought about an immense reduction in the amount of disease and suffering; not, of course, in isolation, but hand in hand with the advancement of science on all fronts, a steadily rising standard of living and a host of public health measures. The infectious diseases are largely controlled, whole areas are free from malaria, smallpox and cholera. Infant and maternal mortality have been brought down to a low level, particularly in the affluent countries, and longevity has been increased. But in spite of all this we do not regard ourselves as being particularly happy or healthy. We are still afflicted by numerous complaints, some of which, like rheumatism and the neuroses, detract from a full enjoyment of life while others, such as coronary heart disease, shorten it needlessly.

Influenced by the great discoveries of Louis Pasteur and Robert Koch, in the field of bacteriology, we have tended to hold an over-simplified view of disease. Bacteria brought about pneumonia, tuberculosis and cholera. Each disease appeared to have one specific cause and any multifactorial origin of disease was frowned upon. Doctors concentrated on the physical causes of disease to the exclusion of less tangible, less measurable factors such as psychological stress, deprivation and disagreeable physical conditions in the environment.

The unifactorial concept of disease also encouraged a curative, as opposed to a preventive, approach. Find out what is attacking the body or what is missing from it and then kill the offending germ or replace the missing factor – such was the general approach.

Emotional factors in the development of disease have been suspected from earliest recorded times and both physicians and poets have written of illness following on disappointed love, frustration and failure, but until the last few decades we have had no means of measuring the changes associated with such emotions as anger, resentment, frustration and despair, and no scientific way of incriminating these emotional states in the causation of disease. Techniques and tools have now become available for the accurate measurement of the biochemical changes associated with the emotions. We have also become aware of the early stages, or precursors of disease and so we are beginning to see how the changes evoked by prolonged and harmful emotional states lead to ill health.

The aim of this book is to set out in comprehensible terms for the lay reader the findings of modern research on the diseases brought about by stressful experiences, to examine potentially harmful factors in society and the environment, to point out warning signals of impending disease and to determine what preventive action is justified and suitable at this stage of our knowledge; and how we can adjust our working lives, our intimate and social relationships to safeguard ourselves against avoidable disease and promote a state of real well-being. The reader may also be spurred on to demand of the Health Services an emphasis on preventive medicine and of society an adjustment of our working lives to promote health.

The last part of the book is devoted to a practical account, in non-technical terms, of the management of some of the commoner stress linked diseases.

1

*

The Concept of Stress

A GENERATION AGO we used to think of physical illness as being entirely due to inherited factors, bacteria, viruses and a variety of physical and chemical agents. Allergy was well on the map and a good deal of the mechanism of this process was understood, but we were uncertain about the part it played in such diseases as asthma and eczema. Our present concepts on Autoimmunity had not yet been developed and we did not realize that the body could make such blunders as to produce antibodies to destroy its own tissues. There were vast gaps in our knowledge in relation to cancer and to diseases of the arteries, and there still are. Psychiatry was as yet a crude science with little curative ability and the link between emotional stress and physical illness was only vaguely appreciated.

Strangely enough, in spite of our lack of understanding of the causation of so many illnesses, we were largely unaware of our ignorance and there was a mood of self-confidence in the medical profession. If we did not know the answers, these appeared to be just around the corner. This confidence was enhanced by the rapid discovery of the antiseptics and antibiotics. The sulphonamides had just come into use for the treatment of a wide range of infections and we felt we would soon have chemicals to cure cancer, rheumatism and other stubborn diseases. Some of these predictions did come true and chemical substances are helping in such fields as mental disorders and raised blood pressure. But the initial optimism petered out as we realized how much more research was needed before the remaining strongholds of disease could be overcome. There is again a new resurgence of optimism based on our research into stress and psychosomatic disease and it is felt that the groundwork has been laid for an understanding of the diseases of blood vessels, of connective tissue and the allergies, and probably some of this optimism is justified. Cancer alone stands out as the great mystery baffling even the most knowledgeable.

There was, as we have said, an era in which it was fashionable to assign to a disease a specific cause and the multifactorial origin of disease was ridiculed. But many observers were not happy about this outlook. Surely many factors were involved even in the simplest of diseases. Why was it that after the bitter and exhausting First World War an influenza epidemic gripped whole nations and killed even the young? Why was it that psychological stress and malnutrition seemed to encourage illness? So we began to think again of the resistance of the individual to disease and we began to analyse factors in this general concept of resistance, to build a scientific framework and a reliable body of data to replace our previous impressions which rested on folklore and individual experience.

Undoubtedly the Second World War prompted and hastened research into resistance to battle stress in particular, and to stress in general. How did the human body cope with the many assaults upon it? How could it stand up to exposure to cold, heat, fear, intense muscular activity, loss of sleep, wounds and pain? It was this sort of experience which the pioneers of research on stress had in mind.

First we must be clear as to what is meant by stress. To some it means unpleasant factors in the environment, such as described above, which act on the individual. The majority of scientists and doctors, however, think of stress as a reaction of the body to strains placed upon it. Thus any such force or stimulus acting on an object will produce a condition of stress in that object or system. In the following pages, then, harmful or traumatic stimuli will be called stressors or stressful factors. The state of stress in the animal is brought about by these factors and prepares it for action in the face of threat or attack.

Stress has been studied by scientists from many disciplines and each makes contributions in his own special field. It is, however, the cross-fertilization of ideas and co-operation between the disciplines that has resulted in the spectacular advances in this vast subject.

The sciences which are particularly involved are Physiology, Medicine, Psychiatry, the Behavioural Sciences, Sociology, Statistics, Industrial Psychology and Industrial Medicine, Public Health and Epidemiology. The proponents of these disciplines, working in various combinations, have produced a number of Schools studying stress and these will be briefly considered here and discussed in greater detail later on.

Some workers were able to study the effects of emotions on organs in man. In the early part of the nineteenth century an American army surgeon, William Beaumont, pioneered this approach using Alexis St Martin as his subject. In this century Stewart Wolf and Harold G. Wolff[1] found a willing subject in the person of Tom who, as a child of nine, had had a surgical opening made into his stomach as he had damaged his gullet beyond repair and this allowed the lining of that organ to be directly viewed. These famous researches opened the way to similar work on the effect of the emotions on the lungs, the heart and blood vessels, the gut and other areas. This was a field in which the psychiatrists and physicians co-operated, each learning from the other, and the immensely broad science of Psychosomatic Medicine was born.

The next great development in the understanding of stress was the discovery of the Fight/Flight reaction of animals. Walter B. Cannon, an outstanding American physiologist, found that all animals respond in a common manner to threat.[2] They prepare for appropriate action, be it aggression or flight, by the mobilization of the autonomic nervous system and the medulla, or core, of the adrenal glands.

Up to the time of Hans Selye, another physiologist, whose major work on Stress and the General Adaptation Syndrome appeared in 1950,[3] scientists discussed stressful stimuli under separate headings, considering that each stimulus had a specific effect and brought about a specific response. To some extent this is true, and each stimulus, such as cold or heat, will bring about a different and specific defence mechanism. Selye, while accepting the specific effect of each stimulus, nevertheless, discovered that a multitude of different stimuli will also bring into play a group of common responses which he called the General Adaptation Syndrome (GAS). Selye was fortunate in having at his disposal new knowledge of the physiology of the pituitary and adrenal glands and his GAS takes into account the crucial role of hormones produced by those organs. Earlier workers were aware of the existence of only some of these hormones and so their appraisal of the stress reaction was necessarily limited.

Another approach is based on the classical work of the great Russian physiologist Ivan Pavlov. Animals and human beings are born with certain reflexes, such as sucking, crying and walking and they acquire a whole gamut of conditioned reflexes which permit a rapid, useful response to outside stimuli without the need for intervention of higher mental processes and judgement. An animal can be trained to make certain conditioned responses and an experimental situation can be built in which, by frustration of that response, controlled anxiety can be induced and studied. Physiologists, psychiatrists and behavioural scientists have joined together in the study of artificially induced stress situations in man. *The Mastery of Stress* by Daniel H. Funkenstein and his colleagues[4] is one important contribution in this field.

A major advance in the recognition of the influence of traumatic life experiences on disease has come from the joint approach of physician and statistician. At one stroke intuition and folklore, which have always held that traumatic personal experiences lead to illness, have been statistically shown to be correct. Thomas Holmes and Richard Rahe's *Cluster Theory of Illness*[5] is a milestone in the history of the study of stress diseases.

Finally a co-operation between physicians, sociologists, statisticians, epidemiologists and workers in industrial medicine has led to the beginnings of an understanding of stress diseases in the industrial and social setting. A symposium held jointly by the World Health Organization and the University of Uppsala in 1970[6] highlights the valuable pioneer work on these inter-disciplinary groups.

So much for a brief résumé of the many trends in the fascinating exploration of stress and disease. Let us now get down to brass tacks. For those that are interested there follows a short chapter on the anatomy and physiology of the systems and organs mainly involved in the stress disorders. Those who know it all may wish to jump to the following chapter.

2

*

The Main Systems involved in the Stress Reaction

WE HAVE DEFINED STRESS as the response of the body to harmful and threatening forces in the environment. These responses are purposeful and are directed towards the goals of survival and adaptation. In the vast majority of cases the body's efforts to cope are successful and the stress is resolved. Yet failure may take place because of the overwhelming nature of the assault or because of inadequate, excessive or inappropriate responses. To understand the difference between success and failure and to plan measures to avoid the latter we must know something about the body's mechanisms for adaptation. Almost all parts of the body are in some way involved in the stress reaction, but we need only concentrate on those systems which play a primary and vital role. The brain, being the receiver, assessor and co-ordinator of information and the director of our defences must be accepted as the leader of all systems involved in the stress reaction, but we can leave our study of it aside until we come to the chapter on the emotions. This narrows the field to the pituitary-adrenal axis and the autonomic (automatic) nervous system. The former is a grand alliance between a small gland at the base of the brain and two rather bigger glands lying some distance away in the remoteness of the back of the abdomen, yet intimately connected with each other and responding subtly to one another so as to cope with major body stresses. The latter is that extraordinary network of nerves which supervises the activity of most of our body organs without conscious effort on our part.

The Pituitary Gland

The pituitary gland is situated at the base of the brain, lying in a bony pit, covered, but for a small perforation, by a fibrous

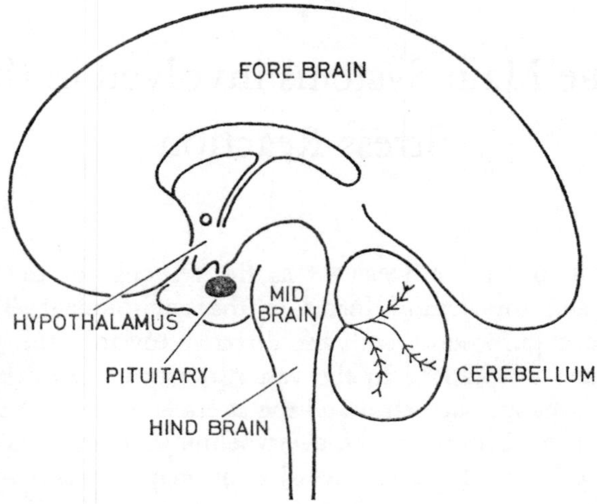

Fig I. Section of brain to show position of the Pituitary Gland

roof. Its highly protected situation is in keeping with its important status. A narrow stalk connects it through the perforation with a portion of the brain called the hypothalamus. The pituitary measures only 12 millimetres across and 8 millimetres from back to front and weighs only half a gram, yet the hormones it produces control a host of important subsidiary glands and its internal structure and functions are a miracle of design and organization. In its turn it is itself controlled by the hypothalamus.

Now a hormone is a 'chemical messenger' produced by an endocrine gland (a gland whose secretions are not channelled away into the gut but are retained in the body) which, when carried by the blood stream to various parts of the body, will have a specific effect on a target organ or target tissues. A good example is insulin which is produced by the pancreatic gland. It enters the blood stream to exert a specific effect on the liver and muscles – the laying down of stores of sugar.

The anterior pituitary is composed of several kinds of cells which can be distinguished by contrasting stains. One small pink staining cell makes Adreno Cortico Trophic Hormone (ACTH), which stimulates the cortex or outer shell of the adrenal gland to produce cortisol – the corner-stone in our resistance to stress. Other cells will, between them, produce six further hormones – those influencing thyroid gland activity, growth, lactation, reproduction and pigmentation of the skin. But, for our purposes, these may be largely disregarded.

ACTH is essential to survival and to the body's ability to cope with stress, so its production must be carefully and accurately controlled to meet exact demands. If too much is produced we have unwanted and serious side effects. If too little, important functions are not maintained. There are two ways in which this hormone is produced. The first by a semi-automatic process, waxing and waning in a natural circadian rhythm (the word circadian meaning 'about twenty-four hours', from the Latin *circa diem*, and it has largely replaced the use of the term diurnal rhythm, which seems to imply day as opposed to day and night rhythm). This rhythmic release of ACTH ensures an adequate level of cortisol in the blood during the early hours of the morning, to cope with the day's work, and a fall in the evening and early part of the night when the resting body makes fewer demands. The second process allows a highly variable output of ACTH and hence of cortisol, in response to fluctuating stress situations as they arise.

There is in addition a self-adjusting negative feedback mechanism in which a raised blood cortisol, the principal hormone of the adrenal cortex, will inhibit ACTH release. This is not, however, the invariable effect of a raised blood cortisol. In times of great stress the negative feedback is put aside and ACTH continues to be produced – as is only logical.

The Hypothalmus serves as a giant switch board, receiving messages from all parts of the body from nerves and through the blood vessels flowing through it. It dispatches messages through the Autonomic Nervous System or by means of Hormones to help the body adapt.[1]

The Adrenal Glands

The two adrenal glands are vital to life. The one on the right has the shape of a cocked hat, that on the left is crescent shaped. They sit on the upper pole of each kidney and thus lie at the back of

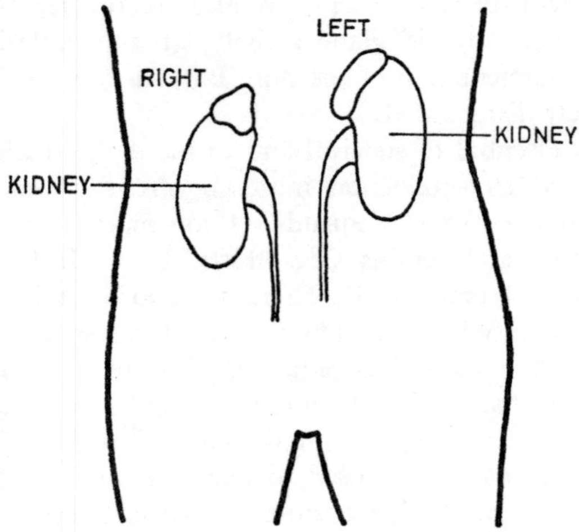

Fig II. The Adrenal Glands

the abdomen behind the peritoneum, a membrane which lines the abdominal cavity. Each gland is about the size of a walnut and weighs 3–4 grams. If cut across it is seen to be made up of two types of tissue. The outer, broader tissue is called the cortex and is yellowish in colour; the inner, narrower one is the medulla and is dark red.

The Adrenal Cortex

The cortex in both men and women, manufactures mainly cortico-steroids (hormones with a chemical structure similar to that of cholesterol and indeed derived from this substance). The medulla produces adrenaline and noradrenaline, which are called epinephrine and norepinephrine in America. Under the microscope the cortex is seen to be composed of three zones. The middle zone contains cholesterol and ascorbic acid (or vitamin C) but only small quantities of cortico-steroids are actually found in any of the zones. This suggests that the cortico-steroids are only produced as the occasion demands and there are no ready stores to be tapped.

There are two main groups of cortico-steroid hormones. The first, the mineralocorticoids, are produced by the cells of the outer zone. As their name implies they control the disposition of salt, potassium and water in the body and so help to regulate the blood pressure. The second group, of even greater importance to us in the context of stress, are the glucocorticoids which are produced by the two inner zones. The main member of this group is cortisol.

In combating stress, adrenaline and noradrenaline, which appear on the scene immediately, are our first vital line of defence but are short lived in action and incapable of sustaining resistance. Cortisol takes longer to come into play, being secreted several minutes after a rise in the blood level of ACTH, but, once on the scene, it will enable prolonged adaptation to stress. Some idea of the time span of its action is given by the finding that blood levels of cortisol will return to normal two to four hours after ACTH has left the blood stream.

How does cortisol help us to adapt to stress? First, it must make available sources of energy. This it does by promoting the production of sugar from stores in the liver (hence the name glucocorticoid), by mobilizing fat from fat depots, and by accelerating the breakdown of protein into simpler components, amino acids, which can be used either as a source of energy or as new building blocks for the repair of damaged tissues. Second, it must prevent excess inflammation and scar tissue formation. When tissues are damaged by harmful agents such as X-rays or chemicals large numbers of cells are killed and to remove these cells and rebuild the tissues the processes of inflammation and repair, by the laying down of scar tissue, are set in motion. Cortisol acts as a watchdog preventing the excess production of inflammatory cells and excess activity of repairing cells. Third, it must counteract shock. In this condition the blood volume drops and with it the blood pressure. Cortisol has a weak mineralocorticoid effect and helps to retain salt and water in the circulation. Finally it must regulate the production of ACTH and this it does by negative feedback control.

Cortisol is produced in stages from cholesterol under the supervision of ACTH and numerous enzymes. It may circulate in the blood as free, active cortisol or may be rendered inactive, till required, by being bound to a blood protein. When no longer needed it undergoes chemical changes in the liver and passes out through the kidney in an inert form.

An unexpected function of cortisol is to counteract a pituitary hormone which induces pigmentation of the skin. In the absence of sufficient cortisol this hormone works overtime and the patient becomes unnaturally and excessively pigmented as is the case in Addison's disease where the adrenal glands have been destroyed. Until the cortisone group of drugs became available this disease was invariably fatal. Life could be maintained for a while in a precarious way by eating large amounts of salt. Later, after Reichstein's classical discovery of DOCA, a mineralocorticoid, the condition could be partly controlled. In the fifties replacement therapy became possible with both glucocorticoids and mineralo-corticoids, and to our intense satisfaction we saw our patients able to lead a normal life. There was, for example, the case of an attractive English woman who returned from a summer holiday apparently splendidly sun tanned. Although she looked well, she felt terribly tired and weak and barely managed to struggle through her daily chores. To her intense surprise the sun tan did not disappear, as it did with everyone else, as autumn and winter passed by. She had indeed developed the pathological pigmentation of Addison's disease. General examination and laboratory tests confirmed the diagnosis. The sugar and salt content of the blood was diminished while that of potassium was increased. Nowadays it is a simple matter to measure the amount of cortisol in the blood and in cases such as this, the level is found to be low; nor can it be raised by an injection of ACTH. The adrenal cortex in health produces some 25 milligrams of cortisol daily and a tenth of a milligram of aldosterone and this is the sort of dose of these two essential cortico-steroids on which the patient was stabilized with excellent results. Requirements of cortisol during stress are greatly increased and patients are instructed to take far larger doses during feverish illnesses and periods of stress.

The Adrenal Medulla

When one looks at the structure of the adrenal medulla one is left in no doubt about its ability to make a rapid contribution in times of stress. Clumps of large cells with particles or granules charged with the precursors of adrenaline and noradrenaline are surrounded by a rich network of blood vessels. In an instant these granules can discharge their contents into the bloodstream.

The proportion of adrenaline to noradrenaline varies in different animal species. The more timorous, such as the rabbit, have a preponderance of adrenaline (some ninety-five per cent), while the more aggressive and robust, like the lion, will produce mainly noradrenaline. In spite of man's reputed tendency to aggression, noradrenaline makes up only about twenty per cent of his medullary hormone output. So perhaps he is not as aggressive as he makes out and will, in time, learn to solve his disputes by non-violent means.

The adrenal medulla is not essential to life but contributes to the animal's greater efficiency under conditions of threat. In the resting dog, a tiny amount of noradrenaline is secreted per minute but this can be increased two hundred fold when the dog is put under great stress, for example on the appearance of a cat.

Muscular exertion, emotional states, pain, suffocation, a drop of blood pressure or of blood sugar and numerous other traumatic influences can bring about an outpouring of adrenaline and noradrenaline which are collectively called catecholamines.

Incoming messages from many parts of the body will act upon an elongated group of nerve cells called the Reticular Formation which stretches from the base of the fore-brain to the hind-brain and this in turn will stimulate the adrenal medulla via the sympathetic nervous system (shortly to be described).

Noradrenaline is not only produced by the adrenal medulla it is also released at the ends of some sympathetic nerve fibres and so it will be seen that the effects of stimulation of the sympathetic nervous system and adrenal gland production of noradrenaline are similar. When the task of these hormones is completed they are inactivated by appropriate enzymes (catalysts formed by living cells) one of which, monoamine oxidase, we will meet again later on in the book as it plays a role in depression.

If we remember that the catecholamines prepare the animal to meet an acute emergency then their actions can be easily understood. Obviously those organs that are essential in times of stress will be alerted, stimulated and better supplied with blood. At the same time inessential organs are allowed to rest and their blood supply is restricted. In other words blood vessels to the heart and muscles are opened up while those supplying the skin and gut are partly shut down. The heart is made to pump out more blood at each stroke and the pulse rate is accelerated. Air intake into the lungs is greatly improved by opening up the small breathing tubes and increasing the rate of respiration. Vision needs to be more sensitive and the pupils enlarge to allow more light to enter. More energy is required so glucose is pushed into the circulation from stores in the liver, and fatty deposits are mobilized and split into easily combustible fatty acids. Digestion can be allowed to rest and the gut becomes idle.

Within a fraction of a second the animal, confronted by an alarming situation, is alerted by catecholamines which have been pumped into the circulation, economies are made wherever possible and energy is diverted to essential organs which are prepared for fight or flight.

As we shall see, the catecholamines are not alone in helping the animal to meet a threat. Their comrade in arms is the sympathetic nervous system. The catecholamines reinforce and prolong the activity of this system.

The Autonomic Nervous System

Our overall nervous system is divided, for convenience, into the central nervous system on the one hand, composed of the brain and spinal cord and, issuing forth from these structures, nerves to the sense organs and limbs and, on the other hand, the autonomic nervous system. The former deals with voluntary conscious effort and reflex activity of our limbs, the latter is concerned with the smooth functioning of our body organs such as heart, lungs and gut and with the correct distribution of blood to these organs and to the limbs. The name given to this second system – autonomic – creates a false impression. It is certainly not autonomous. Indeed it is intimately linked anatomically and functionally with the central nervous system and co-operates with it. It might, more appropriately, be called the 'silent service', unobtrusively controlling the activity of our body organs and performing a host of essential tasks without demanding of us a conscious supervision.

Until recently it was not thought possible to influence bodily functions such as regulation of the pulse rate, blood pressure and the temperature of the limbs by voluntary means. These matters were considered to be the sole province of the autonomic nervous system. We now find, perhaps through the influence of Yoga

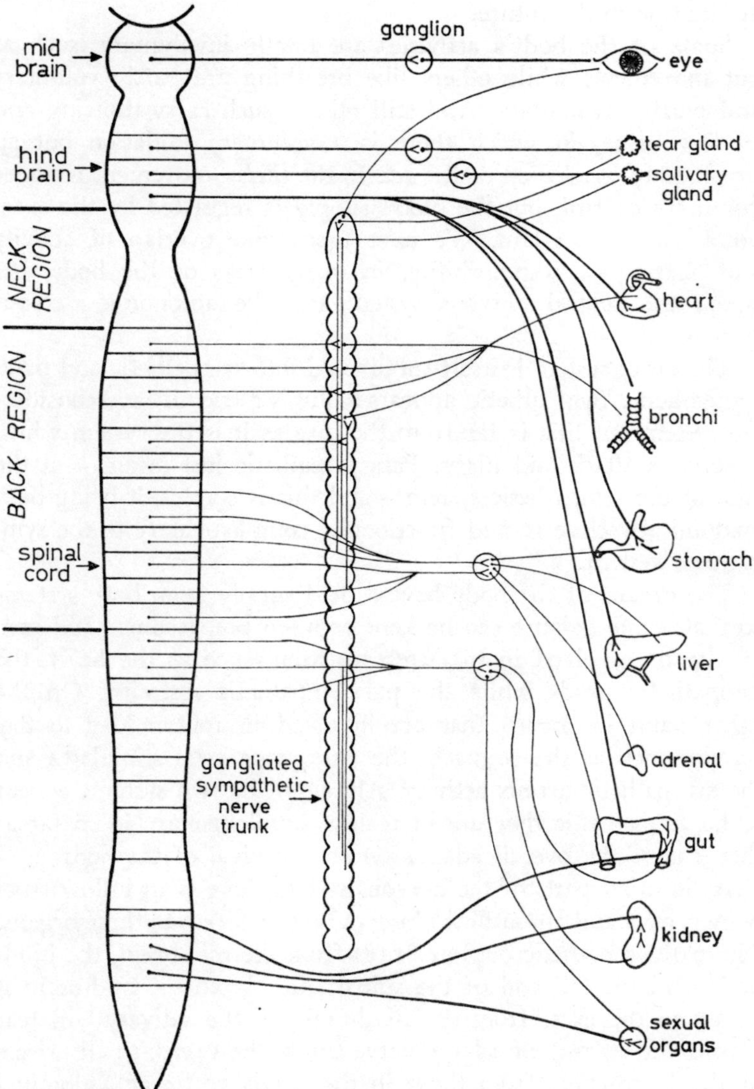

Fig III. The Autonomic Nervous System
Thin lines indicate Sympathetic fibres
Thick lines indicate Parasympathetic fibres

philosophers and teachers, that we can, to a limited extent, learn to influence these activities and this may lead to some therapeutic application in the future.

Some of the body's activities are totally involuntary, such as gut movement, while others like breathing are partly voluntary and partly involuntary. And still others, such as swallowing and passing urine, in which there is a voluntary initiation but an involuntary conclusion of the act. In the limbs, movement is under voluntary control, but the blood supply is regulated by the autonomic nervous system. We have then some overlap of activity and sharing of responsibility, in many areas of the body, between the central nervous system and the autonomic nervous system.

The latter system is itself subdivided into sympathetic and parasympathetic. 'Sympathetic' appears to imply a friendly and considerate system but this is far from the case as it is the system which supervises attack and flight. Parasympathetic just means – at the side of the sympathetic system – and this is correct, it being both anatomically close to and functionally complementary to the sympathetic system.

The organs of the body have a dual supply from both systems so that a fine balance can be kept between preparedness and rest. In organs involved in the stress reaction, such as the heart, the sympathetic prods while the parasympathetic restrains. On the other hand in organs that are involved in routine day to day activity such as the stomach, the parasympathetic stimulates and the sympathetic arrests activity. Although the two systems appear to be antagonistic they are in reality complementary in so far as they ensure the overall adaptation and survival of the body.

As in other parts of the nervous system there is an inflow from body organs and an outflow along outgoing nerves to these organs. The parasympathetic outflow arises from the mid-brain, the hind-brain and the tail end of the spinal cord. From the mid-brain it passes to the eyes, from the hind-brain to the salivary and tear glands and by way of a large nerve trunk, the vagus, to all organs of the body apart from those in the pelvis or lower abdominal cavity lying between the hips. These are supplied by nerves from the terminal part of the cord.

The sympathetic outflow arises from cells in a specialized part of the spinal cord called the lateral column, which extends from the upper chest to the lumber region in the lower back.

The main function of nerve cells in the brain and the spinal cord is that of communication. For this purpose the cell possesses a number of short threads called dendrites to collect information and a long nerve fibre called an axon which transmits information over long distances; for example from the spinal cord to the tips of fingers or toes. Both parasympathetic and sympathetic pathways are served by two relays of nerves. The first consists of nerve cells with long axons which extend for some distance to reach a ganglion or relay post. The second relay nerve cell, situated in the ganglion will carry messages along further axons to their destination in muscle or gland. Electric impulses will pass from the brain or spinal cord along the first relay. At the junction the message is transmitted by a chemical called acetylcholine to the second relay cell. If these be parasympathetic the final message to the organ is again mediated by acetylcholine. At the terminals of sympathetic nerves adrenaline or noradrenaline are produced to stimulate structures supplied by these nerves. There is one exception to this. Sweat glands which are supplied by sympathetic fibres are nonetheless stimulated by acetylcholine.

The sphere of influence of any one parasympathetic nerve tends to be localised and more discrete, while sympathetic activity is usually far more diffuse, and this is understandable, as it is the messenger for action and many parts of the body require immediate and simultaneous preparation. To achieve this type of reaction the sympathetic outflow passes from the segments of the spinal cord to two long gangliated nerve trunks, lying on each side of the spinal column, which may be compared to motorways and permit unhindered traffic up and down their whole length. As in a motorway there are convenient access points in the shape of white and grey communicating paths.

The peripheral autonomic nervous system is influenced by activities at higher levels in the brain and brain stem and especially by the brain stem reticular formation, various aggregations of cells such as the thalamic nucleus and hypothalamus and numerous ascending and descending pathways connecting these regions.

With the help of the endocrine system the autonomic nervous system controls a vast empire of body organs so efficiently and quickly that we are for long stretches of time unaware of that part of our existence. The parasympathetic carries out a number of functions which are needed when the body is resting or is not required to make a special effort. It brings about contraction of the pupil and secretion of saliva. It slows the heart rate, constricts the breathing tubes, relaxes the circular valves of the gut and bladder, opens up capillary vessels in the skin and bowel. It takes part in sexual activity and induces dilatation of the blood vessels of the erectile tissue of the penis and clitoris.

The actions of the sympathetic nervous system are almost identical with those of the catecholamines and serve to mobilize the full resources of the body in times of activity and combat. Perhaps we should just add that the sympathetic system causes secretion of sweat glands and erection of the hairs in the skin which remind us that we are very much part of the animal world.

3

*

Walter B. Cannon
The Fight or Flight Response

WALTER B. CANNON, who was born in Wisconsin, United States of America, in the eighteen seventies, was one of those marvellous men who combined in one person the talents of physician, physiologist, philosopher and readable writer.

Charles Darwin had shown that man was the culmination of a long evolutionary process and contained in his body the structures common to the animal world. Cannon in turn showed that man had a common functional organization with animals which gave him the power to survive in a hostile, competitive and threatening world. In his numerous researches he described the resources which are available in times of threat, the ways in which they are mobilized and the efficiency and rapidity of the mechanisms involved. He was mainly concerned with the advantages of this mechanism for survival but he also considered the possibility that it could have adverse effects and that these might lead to disease.

By chance Cannon lived for a time in that part of Wisconsin where, in the eighteen thirties, Dr William Beaumont, described by Sir William Osler as the 'Pioneer American Physiologist', had worked in an army outpost and had carried out, without formal training or special equipment, some of the most interesting early research on the effect of the emotions on digestion. Beaumont had been fortunate in coming across a soldier wounded in the abdomen and who, in consequence, had a direct opening to his stomach. He did not let this unique opportunity pass and the man, Alexis St Martin was persuaded to submit to various observations on his gastric secretion and movement over a period of many years. It may be that these studies of Beaumont's, which were so accurately and truthfully recorded, stimulated Cannon into research of a similar kind. We know that in 1896 Cannon, then only a first year medical student, carried out research on the mechanism of swallowing, using the newly developed X-rays to follow opaque material down the long neck of a goose. He extended Beaumont's studies on hunger, thirst and the influence of various emotions on the process of digestion and was eventually led into work of a wider nature in which he considered the significance of the major emotions and their effects on adaptive processes in the body. His widely acclaimed book – *Bodily Changes in Pain, Hunger, Fear and Rage* was first published in 1915 and brought up to date in 1929.[1] Cannon quotes William Harvey, physician and discoverer of the circulation, and the eminent physiologist Ernest Starling as his philosophical guides. The former had written 'Study out the Secrets of Nature by way of experiment'. While the latter, in a preface to a lecture given in 1923 had said 'only by understanding the wisdom of the body shall we attain that mastery of disease and pain which will enable us to relieve the burden of mankind'.

Cannon came to the conclusion as a result of his observations that the major emotions of rage, pain and fear found their outlet mainly through sympathetic activity, while the lesser emotions, which are part and parcel of daily living, such as satisfaction and aversion were mediated by the parasympathetic. There was no strict dividing line and a minor emotion might become overwhelming and express itself through the sympathetic. By and large the sympathetic was concerned with defence and aggression, the parasympathetic with routine bodily activity including nutrition and the conservation of resources for anticipated emergencies. In times of peace a community will devote its energies to mundane processes, to the accumulation of wealth, to the arts and social pleasures. But if an emergency should arise, if, for example, war is declared, these quiet processes are put aside and all the energies of the community are devoted to survival. This is an apt analogy to the relationship between the sympathetic and the parasympathetic. If there is a state of alarm then the calm bodily processes, dealing with such matters as the absorption of food are all stopped abruptly and the sympathetic takes over and puts the body into a state of alert.

This is well illustrated in the process of gastric secretion and movement. Pleasurable experiences and emotions aid these processes while unpleasant emotions put an end to them. Ivan Pavlov had shown this in dogs in whom he had produced a separate gastric pouch and a gullet opening onto the neck. By this means they could be subjected to sham feeding. They derived satisfaction from chewing and swallowing and, even though food did not enter their stomachs, gastric secretion took place after five minutes and continued for a while after feeding was stopped. The sight and smell of food would provoke both a secretion of saliva and gastric juice. We all know how the mouth waters in anticipation of a good meal. There is then a 'psychic secretion' not due to food itself but due to the pleasurable anticipation of food.

In 1878, Charles Richet had made a similar observation on a girl whose gullet had been accidentally damaged and obstructed, so that she had to have an artificial opening made into her stomach. When she chewed tasty food which she could not in fact swallow, gastric secretion would take place. If the food was tasteless this secretion did not occur. Unpleasant emotions will inhibit the flow of saliva, of gastric juices and even, so it was found by later experiments, of bile and pancreatic juices.

Sham feeding in dogs will bring about gastric secretion but this is immediately halted when the dog is disturbed by a cat.

Cannon describes the ancient Indian custom, long superseded by the due processes of the law, when suspected criminals were tried by the 'Ordeal of Rice'. A portion of sacred rice would be given to the suspected persons. After a time they were asked to spit out the morsel of rice on to a leaf. He whose rice had remained dry, was judged to be guilty. Only in him would high excitement inhibit the flow of saliva.

Further experiments showed that the principles which apply to secretion are also valid as far as movement of the gut is concerned. The sight of desirable food or pleasurable feeding will initiate contraction of the stomach and intestines. Constriction of the gut is partly an inherent property and can take place in the absence of the parasympathetic, in this case vagal, activity; however cutting the vagus will abolish movement brought about by psychic stimuli. Nowadays a vagotomy, or section of the appropriate fibres of the vagus, is carried out on patients in the treatment of persistent duodenal ulceration. The psychic element of secretion and motility is abolished but gastric emptying still takes place in response to swallowing and distention of the stomach.

Rage and fear will, on the other hand, inhibit movement by stimulation of the sympathetic and discharge of adrenaline, which brings about a contraction of the sphincters, or circular valves, and relaxation of the smooth muscle.

Cannon goes on to consider the effect of fear and anger on other bodily functions. These emotions will give rise to a raised blood sugar and at times a spill-over of sugar into the urine; a shortening of clotting time; an increase in the number of red cells in the circulation by contraction of the spleen and a restoration of function to fatigued muscle. Athletes will often be found to have sugar in the urine after a strenuous match. The effect of adrenaline on fatigued muscle is interesting. If an electrical impulse is passed along a nerve-muscle preparation isolated, let us say, from a frog's leg, the strength of the current after a time becomes inadequate to make the muscle contract. The muscle is fatigued and the threshold at which an electrical impulse will succeed in stimulating it is raised. Rest, by itself, will lower the threshold and restore function in fifteen minutes to two hours while adrenaline will do so in three to five minutes.

What then is the value of these bodily changes to animals? Cannon makes the important point that one must distinguish between the correctness of the data, which few will dispute, and the inferences to be drawn from them which, in some instances, may be the subject of argument. It is fair to assume that the body's reaction to fear and pain are in the nature of reflexes and serve a purpose. The outward response of an animal to rage with baring of the teeth and bristling of the hair serves to terrify its attackers. Tension of the muscles, gnashing of teeth, protrusion of claws, growls and flaring of the nostrils appear to be weaker forms of actions which would be used to kill the prey. These reflexes had been developed over the course of evolution as a means of survival. The animal spurred on by fear may adopt an offensive posture or, if more appropriate, a defensive one, with efforts to hide, trembling and crying.

The reaction to fear is prompt. In ten seconds the heart beat will become rapid and in some three to six minutes the blood sugar rises.

The emotion of pure fear is related to the flight instinct, whereas if fear is turned to anger then this is linked with the pugnacity or aggressive instinct. Pain, a common sequel of an animal's struggle, adds to the strength of his bodily responses. In the words of Charles Darwin:

> In the agony of pain almost every muscle in the body is brought into strong action. Great pain urges all animals, and has urged them through endless generations to make the most violent and diversified efforts to escape from the cause of suffering.

Pain does not invariably lead to favourable bodily responses and Cannon quotes experiments in which a fall of blood pressure was noted, but he does not explain this observation properly. Fear, if it amounts to terror may temporarily paralyse, especially if there is 'no definite deed to perform'.

Partial asphyxia often accompanies great muscular effort and Cannon found it can cause an out-flow of adrenaline and improve performance by mobilizing sugar, opening up the breathing tubes and increasing blood flow to the limbs. He thought that the phenomenon of 'Second Wind', so well known to athletes could be explained on this basis.

Emotional excitement can be viewed as a means of mobilizing energy. In Cannon's words '. . . these changes are directly serviceable in making the organism more effective in the violent display of energy which fear or rage or pain may involve.'

Some interesting historical examples are given of the mass display of energy, endurance and frenzy. In 1374, a mania broke out in Germany, the Netherlands and France. The victims danced in honour of St John, with unimaginable vigour for hour after hour, uttering cries and seeing visions. In 1740 an extraordinary Sect known as the 'Jumpers' arose in Wales. According to John Wesley:

> After the preaching was over any who pleased gave out a verse of a hymn; and this they sung over and over again, with all their might and main, thirty or forty times, till some of them worked themselves into a sort of drunkenness or madness; they were then violently agitated, and leaped up and down in all manner of postures, frequently for hours together.

Dr William Sargant, a leading present-day London psychiatrist, has made similar observations on tribal rituals in many parts of the world in which, by the aid of music and dance, group excitement will lead to prolonged, tireless activities culminating in a trance state.

Where are these emotions located? According to William James and C. Lange who presented their views in 1884 and 1885 respectively, an object stimulates a sense organ, incoming impulses travel to the cortex of the brain and are perceived. Impulses then travel from cortex to muscles and body organs, where complex changes take place. These changes in the bodily state set up stimuli which travel back to the cortex so that the 'Object – simply – apprehended' becomes the 'Object – emotionally – felt'. In other words emotional colouring is given to impressions by affected parts of the body and its organs, but mainly by the latter. The emotions, according to this theory, are peripheral. Cannon contradicts these arguments and asserts that the seat of emotions is in the thalamus, situated in the posterior half of the ancient fore brain. An animal which has lost its cerebral cortex and the front half of this older fore brain is capable of all the expressions of fear and rage, both in the form of display and the bodily adjustments which are called for.

In the human being the cerebral cortex can inhibit or modify the expression of the emotions, at least in their outward display. If, however, emotion is very strongly felt it can burst through the barrier of inhibition and we find we cannot restrain laughter or anger. If the cortex, or communications to the cortex are damaged on one side, as may be the case in a 'stroke', voluntary movement of the other side of the face becomes impossible. Laughter, however, can be expressed on both sides, even the paralysed one. In the condition of pseudo-bulbar palsy, where tracts between the thalamus and cortex are damaged and both sides of the face are to some degree paralysed, the patient breaks out in uncontrolled fits of laughter and crying. The inhibitory influence of the cortex is absent. And again, there are cases in which the thalamic nuclei are damaged on both sides in which voluntary movement of the face is possible but spontaneous laughter does not take place.

Although the cerebral cortex can usually suppress outward expression of emotion it cannot suppress the inward effects; and visceral changes will continue if the emotions have been roused.

We ought now to return to the emotional derangements of bodily functions. Cannon realized that strong emotions had a survival value even though not all their effects were on the credit side. It was common knowledge, and examples were presented in the medical literature, that emotional crises could be followed by disease or even death. Cannon's views on emotional derangements in some ways anticipated the later work of Hans Selye, who believed that a derailment of the 'General Adaptation Syndrome' could lead to a specific group of diseases. We shall come to that subject in the next chapter.

Cannon was, of course, mainly concerned with the physiology of conflict, but he recognized that physiological (normal) changes could move 'towards the pathological' (abnormal) and that the function of an organ could be so altered that it might fail to perform its customary task. For example he envisaged that the kidney might be damaged in response to excessive stimulation and fail to get rid of waste, thus poisoning the whole body. He was aware also that bodily change in response to emotion may become so persistent as to become a menace instead of a benefit.

He considered some concrete examples of illness resulting from emotional situations. His own work on the effect of the emotions on the digestive tract pointed to the possibility of cessation of secretion and motility in cases of fear and anxiety, and many examples were available in the literature of patients who had stopped eating, or who suffered from persistent vomiting after some frightening experience and were cured by the relief of fear.

During the First World War a condition called 'Soldiers Heart' or 'Disorderly action of the Heart' was common in shell shocked soldiers. It was reasonable to suppose that the stresses of war had sensitized the sympathetic control of the heart so that the slightest excitement would result in a rapid pulse, discomfort in the chest and even shortness of breath.

Foster gave a fascinating report in 1927 which illustrated the mechanism of this type of disorder. In brief, the circumstances were as follows. A wife, known to be free of heart disease saw her husband arm in arm with another woman in the street. She fled home in distress and stayed there for several days. When, later, she attempted to go out, she feared to meet her rival and put off the ordeal. Eventually she determined to go out and found that her heart thumped rapidly, she felt an oppression in the chest and a choking sensation in the throat and had to return home. This happened every time she tried to go out. She felt she might die in the street. Yet no organic disease of the heart could be found. By a process of conditioning and association some trivial stimulus could bring about a return of the distress, and the accompanying bodily changes which she had felt in that first unhappy moment.

High blood pressure, in Cannon's view, could be linked with increased sympathetic activity.

Thyroid overactivity had often been found to follow emotional trauma. A striking case of Emerson's is quoted in a married woman with two illegitimate children whose husband committed suicide in her presence as a rebuke. Six weeks later she had developed Grave's Disease in which the thyroid gland is overactive and enlarged. In considering this particular case doctors would now after several more decades of research have considerable misgivings. The facts were correct enough, but the inference that sympathetic overactivity was the cause of the disease would now be questioned.

The next problem was how derangement of bodily processes were brought about by emotion. Cannon quotes the work of Watson on infants. This investigator found that, from the beginning, loud sounds and indications of loss of support were the natural stimuli for fear, and that hampering of freedom of bodily movement is the natural stimulus for rage. There is the question of interpretation of a stimulus. This is the province of the cerebral cortex. We might be frightened by a real bear but not by a stuffed one. The cortex will discriminate and influence the older forebrain.

In the normal physiological response to fear there is visceral activity, the animal overcomes the threat by combat or flight and the situation is resolved. In the pathological response the stimulus may persist and the reflex activity likewise continues. In some cases resolution is not possible. In the case where, for example, the husband committed suicide in his wife's presence 'Nothing could be done. The acts were final. They could not be forgotten. Many associations recalled them'.

The work of Pavlov had greatly helped our understanding of the development of harmful habits and processes. He had shown how an indifferent stimulus could become an effective conditioning stimulus. Saliva will flow if a dog is shown food. If then an indifferent stimulus such as a red light be repeatedly added to the natural stimulus the dog will learn to salivate when shown the red light by itself. The reflex has become a conditioned reflex. Any indifferent stimulus can become a conditioning stimulus. The process is carried out in the cerebral cortex.

In this way a baby who may play fearlessly with a white rat can become adversely conditioned to be afraid of it by linking the presence of the white rat repeatedly with a loud, unpleasant noise. The white rat becomes a conditioned stimulus and the baby will cry when presented with it. It has become the symbol of something frightening.

Many stimuli, which in themselves are harmless, may then become unpleasant by association and memory and so 'the persistent derangements of bodily function in strong emotional reactions can be interpreted as due to the persistence of the stimuli which evoke the reactions'.

It is worth quoting Cannon when he gives his reasons for dwelling on the physiological mechanisms of emotional disturbances. He gives two main reasons. 'First I wished to show that these remarkable perturbations could be described in terms of neurone processes. And, again, I wished to show that these interesting phenomena need not be set aside as mystical events occurring in the realm of the Psyche.'

Cannon was critical of the approach of many physicians to emotional bodily disturbances. He thought they tended to avoid these patients. Firstly because there was no recognized pathology and secondly because they fell into the category of disturbance of the 'Psyche', which was no concern of theirs. He was therefore not surprised that the sufferers turned, in their despair, to faith healers. Obviously Cannon thought physicians should understand the physiological basis of these conditions and should accept responsibility for them. His viewpoint has been vindicated.

He made some practical suggestions on the management of diseases brought about by the emotions: that treatment should be offered early before the processes become deep set in the neural organization.

It should be understood that it was not possible 'to argue' a patient out of his fears. After all the condition was largely subcortical. The fear must be genuinely removed or explained. He advocated avoidance of noxious stimuli.

Conditioned stimuli could be inhibited by introduction of new and unusual stimuli. Perhaps he was thinking of desensitization, which is now practised.

Where the reason for the disturbance was not clear he advocated careful enquiry or analysis. If the origin of the disturbance could be brought to light a cure would often follow.

Finally, he gave a word of warning that it was dangerous to assume that all forms of disease, where there was no obvious organic cause, were due to emotional factors. One should not fail to look carefully for organic pathology. It was all very sound advice.

In assessing the contribution which Cannon has made to the understanding of the diseases of stress, one has to remember that his main work was done half a century ago. Noradrenaline had not yet been discovered. Some of the activities which Cannon claimed for adrenaline are in fact brought about by noradrenaline, but the difference in action between these two substances is not very striking and does not alter the main conclusions of Cannon's work. The existence of Cortisol had not yet been realized so that some of the bodily changes which he had ascribed to adrenaline were in fact brought about by cortisol either alone, or acting in a complementary fashion to adrenaline. For example the rise in blood sugar in response to emotion or pain is only partly brought about by adrenaline. Cortisol is responsible for some of the rise. The origin of many diseases was less clear than it is now. Given these factors one can only be astonished at the extent of his achievements. By making clear the physiology of the animal's power to adapt to outside threats, he helped to establish a base on which further work could be done. He realized that numerous external and internal stimuli (pain after all is an internal stimulus) which we would now call stressors, have something in common – a threat to survival, and that there is a common mechanism by which they influence the body, this being the Autonomic Nervous System and the adrenal medulla. True, he considered that this mechanism was almost the whole of our defence and he was unaware of the value of the adrenal cortex, which is our second, and more persistent line of defence. But his concept of the Fight or Flight reaction as a complex reflex response conditioned by cortical assessment and supervision, was correct and remains a valid one.

Some of his inferences were, in the light of further knowledge, wrong and he was well aware of this possibility. It is, for example, unlikely that sympathetic overstimulation plays a significant role in chronic thyroid overactivity. The auto-immune basis of the disease in most patients was then unknown and could not have been suspected. The fall in blood pressure which he had noted in some forms of pain may perhaps be better explained as due to tissue damage and shock. When he discusses diseases of the alimentary tract, he naturally concentrates on the role of the sympathetic and parasympathetic ignoring many other possible causative factors. It must, however, be admitted that we still do not know the cause of such apparently simple conditions as stomach ulcers. It is remarkable how few errors there were in Cannon's conclusions and we think he must be ranked as one of the great men of science and medicine who have advanced our knowledge of stress enormously. Above all he has given us a rational approach to this subject based on experiment.

4

*

Hans Selye
Adaptation and Disease

THE NAME OF HANS SELYE, has been a byword in Medicine ever since his famous General Adaptation Syndrome (GAS) appeared on the scene in 1936 in the form of a letter to *Nature* called 'A syndrome produced by diverse nocuous agents.'[1]

Many doctors welcomed his work enthusiastically, considering that it opened up a new chapter in medicine, linking stressful experiences, in a scientific way, with disease. On the other hand many others attacked him bitterly for conjuring up complicated and fanciful theories, developed through animal experiments, and applying these without justification to man. His numerous animal experiments were, he claimed, carefully recorded and could be repeated by any other scientific worker. The results of these experiments must be accepted as accurate. A general concept of the body's reaction to stress emerged and that too was widely accepted. He made only tentative hypotheses when considering the relationship of stress to human disease. In his view a derailment of the GAS could result in various diseases but further work was needed to supply more evidence and finally, proof.

Selye's GAS might be considered as a sophisticated elaboration of Cannon's Concept in which the animal responds to outside threat by the immediate involvement of the autonomic nervous system and the adrenal medulla. Cannon had established that there was an element of uniformity in resistance to stress. Selye carried these ideas further by including the pituitary-adrenal axis in the overall design, by describing in great detail the chemical processes involved in the reaction and by dividing the adaptation syndrome into three logical stages progressing from alarm to resistance and finally, in some cases, to exhaustion or failure. In addition he made a more comprehensive attempt at linking disease with faulty adaptational responses.

The GAS may be summarized as follows. When animals are subjected to a variety of stressors with widely differing characteristics there are two types of reaction. The first, a specific reaction in response to the special properties of the stressor and the second, a common, non-specific, reaction independent of the nature of the stressor. The reactions take place concurrently. If, for example, we take cold as a stressor, the animal will display a specific reaction to counteract this stimulus – namely action to prevent heat loss and shivering, and a non-specific reaction which Selye calls the GAS. Some other examples of stressors are painful stimuli, X-rays, ultra-violet light, burns, haemorrhage and asphyxia.

The whole syndrome is divided into three phases. That of the alarm reaction (itself composed of short lived stages of shock and countershock), the stage of resistance, and the stage of exhaustion.

When there is injury of any sort to parts of the body there will be a phase of shock which is characterized by a drop of temperature and blood pressure, by increased capillary permeability and seepage of fluid out of the blood stream with concentration of the blood. There will be tissue breakdown and small ulcers may form in the gut. This phase seems to contain little of positive value to the animal and, indeed, shows all the signs of damage.

It is not until the phase of countershock that we see an effort to correct the damage and restore homeostasis or the condition of normality. In this phase it is apparent that the body makes efforts to regain control. The adrenal cortex enlarges and there is a reversal of the changes seen in shock.

As the stressful stimulus continues and the animal adapts itself, it enters the stage of resistance. The temperature and blood pressure return to normal. Excess breakdown products such as lactic acid are removed from the blood stream. Blood sugar rises again and stays at a slightly elevated level. Blood chlorides, which had dropped in the stage of shock, return to normal. The adrenal cortex is widened and shows signs of activity. The animal is able to cope with the heavier demands made on it and yet maintain its normal, physiological internal environment.

At this point all may be well, the stressor may be removed and normality regained or the state of stress may remorselessly continue till adaptation breaks down. A state of exhaustion sets in with a return of all the ingredients of shock. Blood pressure and tem-

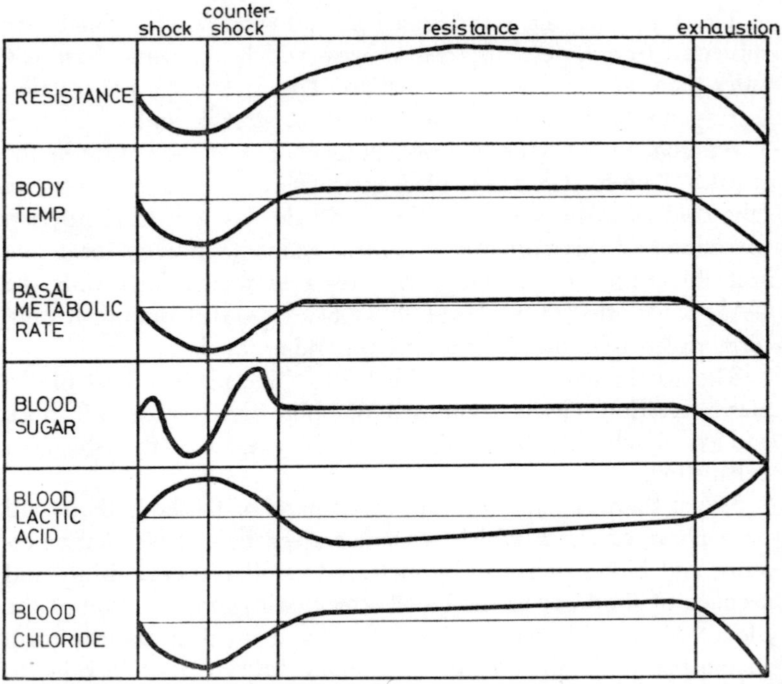

Fig IV. Graphic summary of some of the processes of the General Adaptation Syndrome

perature fall once more. Blood chlorides and blood sugar dip down again. The level of breakdown products in the blood rises. The adrenals show widespread damage to the cortex and obvious loss of function. Death ensues. Some of these processes are dramatically illustrated by a selection of graphs from one of Selye's books (Fig. IV).

Selye discusses the pathways and mechanisms through which stress elicits the bodily reactions described above (Fig. V).

The stressor acts on some part of the body causing local tissue damage which will bring about shock on the one hand and defence on the other. The nervous component of defence acts through the hypothalamus which in turn initiates activity of the autonomic nervous system and the adrenal medulla. There is also hormonal defence which is likewise mediated by the hypothalamus. The pituitary is made to pour out more ACTH and this stimulates the

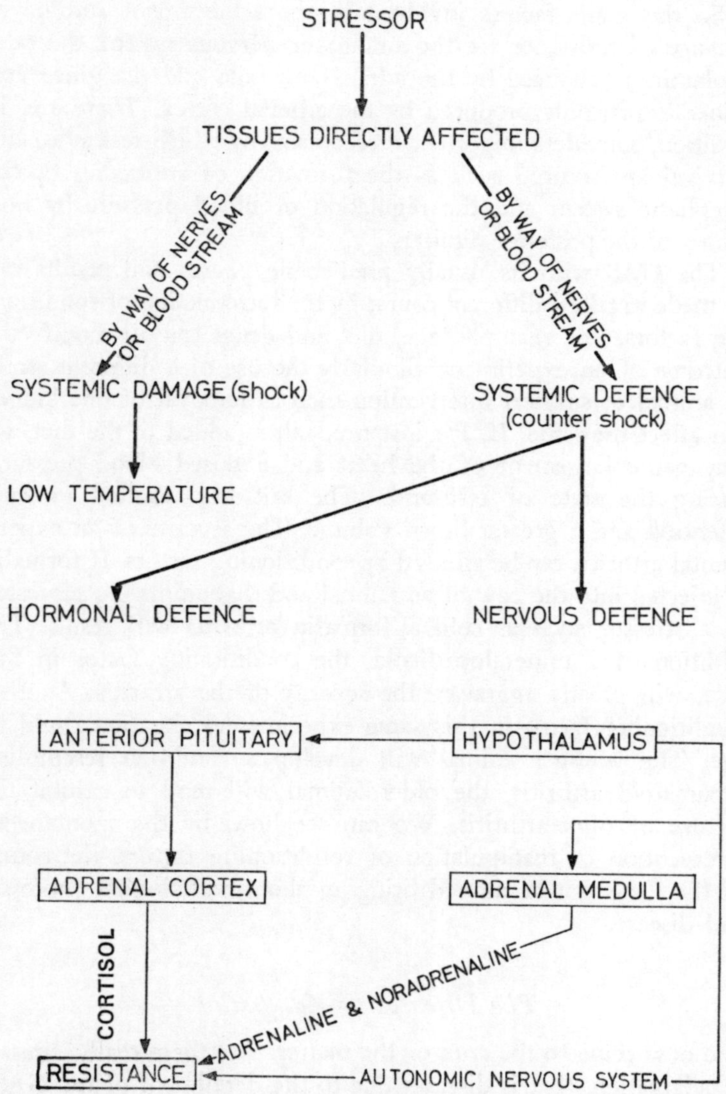

Fig V. Pathways through which stress elicits systemic (bodily) reactions

adrenal cortex to mobilize gluco and mineralocorticoids to bolster up defence.

So the main factors involved in the achievement and maintenance of resistance are the autonomic nervous system, the catecholamines produced by the adrenal medulla and the gluco and mineralocorticoids produced by the adrenal cortex. There are, in addition, some less important mechanisms by which resistance and survival are secured such as the formation of antibodies by the lymphatic system and the regulation of blood pressure by hormones of the posterior pituitary.

The GAS with its usually predictable phases and results can be made to take a different course by the introduction of conditioning factors. For example, age, diet and drugs can all modify the outcome of an experiment. Similarly the use of a different strain of animal or surgical intervention such as removal of one kidney can affect the issue. If, for instance, salt is added to the diet, we may get enlargement of the heart and a raised blood pressure, during the state of resistance. The salt has resulted in fluid retention and a greater blood volume. The severity of an experimental arthritis can be affected by conditioning factors. If formalin is injected into the paw of an animal and that animal be subjected to a stressor such as cold a formalin arthritis will result. The addition of a mineralocorticoid, the conditioning factor in this case, will greatly aggravate the severity of the arthritis. Another conditioning factor in this same experimental situation could be age. The younger animal will develop a condition resembling rheumatoid arthritis, the older animal will tend to exhibit the picture of osteo-arthritis. We can see how, by the spontaneous intervention or manipulation of conditioning factors, the course of the GAS can be altered bringing about pathological processes and disease.

The Diseases of Adaptation

We now come to the crux of the matter. Are there really diseases of adaptation, that is diseases due to the derailment of the GAS? Selye considers there are and classifies them into diseases of overactivity and abnormal activity of the organs of adaptation on the one hand and underactivity of these organs on the other. Overactivity might be due to growths or cancers of the pituitary or adrenal glands or to excessive response of these organs to stresses. We would question the inclusion of these cancers as the predominant factor is a tumour and not necessarily a disease of stress. In the second group, that of secondary overactivity, he places a number of diverse diseases such as high blood pressure, the rheumatic diseases and some psychosomatic diseases. It is this group which is of particular interest to us. The diseases of underactivity again include primary conditions of the pituitary and adrenal glands in which destruction leads to failure and a secondary inadequacy by reason of insufficient response during a stress reaction. Into this last group are placed some infrequent and unimportant conditions such as acute ulcers of the gut. We shall see shortly that this general classification is unlikely to stand up to close examination and further experiment. For example, conditions such as the rheumatic diseases will probably need to be transferred from the overactivity to the underactivity group.

Selye found that he could induce an inflammatory effect in experimental animals by the use of mineralocorticoids. So he called these hormones prophlogistic (borrowing an eighteenth-century word 'phlogistic' which denoted something combustible or inflammatory). The prophlogistic corticoids or PCs would increase infiltration of tissues by inflammatory white cells and encourage deposition of connective or scar tissue. Glucocorticoids on the other hand had an anti-inflammatory effect and these he called antiphlogistic corticoids or ACs. In Selye's view excess of PCs could lead to a raised blood pressure by causing salt retention and to rheumatic disorders by means of their inflammatory properties. He contrived a complex experiment on rats, involving the manipulation of several conditioning factors, to demonstrate his case. One kidney was removed, mineralocorticoids were administered and the animals were fed a high salt diet. Finally they were subjected to cold. They developed high blood pressure, disease in the remaining kidney and transient arthritis.

Can these animal experiments be accepted as evidence that similar pathological changes can occur in man under stress? The arguments for and against Selye's views are extremely complicated. We would say that the balance of opinion is that he is less right than wrong. In the case of raised blood pressure there is some evidence to support excess production of mineralocorticoids as part of the mechanism. But when we come to the rheumatic or connective tissue diseases few doctors would agree with Selye's views. One of the best reviews of the subject is by Walter Bauer and William S. Clark.[2] These authors agree that some forms of emotional and physical stress often play a part in the onset of connective tissue disease. However there is no evidence of a preponderance of mineralocorticoid production through derangement of the pituitary-adrenal axis in the rheumatic diseases. In fact rheumatoid arthritis may take place even in the absence of a functioning pituitary or adrenal gland as, for example, in Addison's disease. Nor do mineralocorticoids, given therapeutically, aggravate this condition.

The final word on all these problems has, however, not been said, as the exact cause or causes of the connective tissue diseases, hypertension and other conditions in Selye's list of diseases of adaptation have not been fully established.

In view of the paucity of support for Selye's clinical conclusions why then do many still regard his work to be of major importance? We think it is because he was able to gather together many threads of the story of stress and weave them into a logical and comprehensive fabric. He has made us aware of the importance of non-specific stressors which will set in motion a fairly uniform type of defensive response. He concentrated attention on the vital role of the pituitary and the adrenal glands in stress and although the diseases of adaptation may not be produced by the exact mechanisms he has outlined, nevertheless many are convinced that the pituitary-adrenal axis plays an important role in these conditions.

Let us quote *some* of the passages from an article written by Selye himself.[3]

> It has been a major endeavour of our Institute to prove that hormones can play a decisive role in the development of several non-endocrine diseases, that is, of maladies which are not primarily due to derangements originating in the endocrine glands themselves.

> The body reacts in a stereotyped manner to a variety of stressors, by the secretion of ACTH and corticoids. Although these help the body to survive during an emergency they may at the same time be harmful. For example, enhance the spread of infection or produce peptic ulcers.

> In the supposed Diseases of Adaptation in man, marked changes in

> the blood level or urinary elimination of hormones can rarely be observed. This fact led to the conclusion that endocrine factors do not play a decisive role in the pathogenesis [origin] of such maladies. However the theory of the Diseases of Adaptation does not postulate an absolute increase or decrease in hormone production, but rather a change in hormone activity. The latter may be due to faulty conditioning, and hence, need not be reflected by any absolute change in hormone level. Thus, a nearly 'normal' glucocorticoid secretion, such as suffices to maintain homeostasis [internal stability] at rest, is grossly insufficient to maintain the life of an animal exposed to stress. Such a hormone secretion also fails to prevent inflammation in the presence of a special irritant e.g. formalin in the case of experimental arthritis. . . .

Many of Selye's arguments are persuasive and logical. Time will tell what contribution he has made to the riddle of 'The Diseases of Adaptation'.

5

*

Psychosomatic Medicine

HAVING LOOKED BACK at the experimental work on stress in animals by Cannon and Selye, we can now continue the story in the human field. Although it has been useful to study the effects of the severe stressors on animals, we can see at once that the stressors with which we have to cope are, on the whole, of a milder and subtler kind. On reaching our office or factory we will not be faced by a ferocious opponent challenging us to physical combat. It is not a cat and dog, or hunter and hunted situation. To be sure there are rivalries and antagonisms but of a controlled kind with limits set by long established custom. Nor are we going to be subjected, apart from episodes of war, to physical mutilation, overexposure to radiation or the extremes of heat and cold. How applicable then are the concepts of the Flight/Fight response of Cannon and the General Adaptation Syndrome (GAS) of Selye to the human scene? The former response is undoubtedly valid, for in the course of our lives we are constantly exposed to situations giving rise to anger and fear of sufficient degree to arouse the Sympathetic System to considerable activity.

We are on less certain ground when we try to apply the knowledge gained from a study of the GAS to human diseases of stress or adaptation. The Alarm Reaction and the Stage of Exhaustion seem to have no human counterpart. Most doctors would, however, if they considered the matter, accept a state equivalent to the Stage of Resistance in human disease. It is, after all, common knowledge that a variety of stressors cause a rise in plasma cortisol and the associated bodily changes which one would expect from this rise. We would subscribe to Selye's idea of the derailment of the GAS, with disease taking place in response to over or underactivity of the organs of adaptation; not hook, line and sinker but with modifications. In addition, it should be noted that Selye's concept takes account of all types of stressors, both physical and mental, and this is important for we should never neglect physical factors.

For some reason overwork and loss of sleep are not given their due emphasis in the causation of illness. They may be accepted as contributory factors in Industrial Fatigue but they are not taken seriously in the disease process. Also forgotten are pleasurable activities which we are accustomed to look upon as entirely beneficial. Unfortunately they too, if intense and prolonged, are under suspicion of being in the category of stressors. If we look at human stress, especially in the urban setting of the developed countries, we will probably agree that its major component is psychological. Here we find overcrowding, noise, competition and conflict and as an outcome of this turbulent environment we suffer from anxiety, frustration, fear and hostility. Let us then, for the moment, perhaps not unreasonably, assume that psychological factors are predominant in the causation of the stress diseases. This leads us to the subject of Psychosomatic Medicine, a term which links the psyche or mind with the soma or body. Psychosomatic diseases may be regarded as physical diseases in whose onset or maintenance mental processes have played an important part. For many years only a handful of diseases were considered truly psychosomatic. The list ran somewhat as follows – asthma, peptic ulcer, rheumatoid arthritis, ulcerative colitis, high blood pressure, overactive thyroid, some connective tissue diseases and some skin disorders. One could add drug addiction, alcoholism and obesity, but these have a less well defined and less constant physical pathology. If however, one thinks in terms of Psychosomatic Medicine then one has to admit that a mental element enters into most illness – indeed some physicians seek to abolish the dividing line between psychosomatic and other diseases and would like us all to become aware of the mental element in the whole spectrum of disease, paying more attention where mental processes predominate. This approach is in keeping with a view expressed many years ago by Professor Adrian, the eminent physiologist, when he gave a lecture on the Mind-Body relationship and made it clear that the mind cannot be separated from the body. His argument went like this: – all sensory input from the environment and from our own bodies reaches us via sensory nerve endings and organs of sensation. The incoming stimuli either set up direct reflex responses or are processed by the brain. There is an appraisal, followed by an emotional or intellectual response, or a mixed response, and later by action if this should be required. The response may be involuntary, ie arousal of the autonomic nervous system and endocrine system, or voluntary in the form of speech or movement. Involuntary and voluntary action may take place concurrently.

Thus it is difficult to conceive of any experience which is purely mental or purely physical. Whatever physical activity we engage in, whether it be work, play, eating or suffering symptoms of illness, there is bound to be a concurrent mental experience; and whatever our mental activity may be there will be a physical component, for even dreaming involves physical activity of brain cells. Moreover some emotional reaction will enter into the most abstract mental process, even if it should be only boredom!

On this analogy we must conclude that a psychological component plays a part in the origin of even the most somatic of diseases. An exception may be a bodily injury in which negligence on the part of the injured had not occurred. Yet physical injury is often due to preoccupation, distraction or lack of concentration and in these cases the existence of an emotional or mental component can scarcely be denied. In bacterial infection, such as an abscess or pneumonia, it is quite probable that worry, insomnia or some other mental strain has weakened the resistance and permitted the infection to take over. Cancer is often regarded as a purely physical disease, yet one Russian research worker has shown that the incidence of skin cancer in rats painted daily with a carcinogenic substance, was far higher in those that were exposed to uncertainty and anxiety than those that were placed in an undisturbed environment. And so, as time passes, more diseases, which were previously thought to be mainly organic or somatic, are coming to be regarded as psychosomatic. For example, it has been found that emotional disturbances will affect the level of blood fats and the speed of clotting and this brings coronary thrombosis and some arterial diseases into the orbit of the psychosomatic.

Before describing two psychosomatic diseases in detail we would like to discuss the concepts of psychosomatic specificity and of secondary gain. In the earlier period of psychosomatic medicine psychiatrists and especially analytic psychiatrists dominated this field and, quite naturally, hoped to describe the disease process in mainly psychological terms. They thought different child-parent relationships brought about different personality traits and specific patterns of internal conflict. In later years particular experiences or situations would activate the internal conflict and precipitate an abnormal or excessive response in an organ or system to produce disease. Thus arose the concept of psychosomatic specificity. If we take asthma as our model, we must imagine the infant reacting to the 'Asthma Mother', who is both loving and rejecting, spoiling and domineering. The child develops a 'characteristic' personality profile which is described by Bastiaans and Groen.[1] It is so detailed and complex that we will not set it out in full, but briefly it includes – egocentricity; impatient and impulsive behaviour which becomes domineering and tyrannical in the family circle; a poor capacity for adaptation; difficulty in solving problems by talking things over; great need for love and affection, often hidden by pseudo-indifference, etc. According to these authors the asthmatic finds it difficult to adapt to situations in which he has to submit to an authoritative person for whom he harbours ambivalent feelings of dependence and aggression. He may react by protest or other activity. If, on the other hand, these reactions are inhibited, either by outside discipline or self-control, an inner conflict develops and the patient feels oppressed. The inner tension becomes 'somatized', or expressed physically, in the form of an asthmatic attack.

Franz Alexander and Thomas French,[2] put it in a somewhat different way. They felt the child had a conflict about crying which is inhibited through fear of maternal repudiation.

> Later in life, difficulty in calling mother by crying gives place to difficulty in confiding in an unpredictable mother or mother substitute. These patients have a conflict between their wish to confide and the fear of it. Thus the fear of alienating mother becomes centred on verbal communications, which explains the involvement of respiratory function. Asthmatic attacks can be understood as an inhibition of the expiratory [breathing out] act for communication, either by crying or confession.

In the analytical formulation there is often a reference to sexuality between mother and child which, to the non-analytically trained, is extremely difficult to grasp. French and Alexander state, 'Some mothers react to the first signs of the little child's sexual strivings directed towards them with withdrawal or rejection. Sexual strivings thus become an internal danger that threatens to alienate mother's affection . . .'

As time passed, analysts realized that not everyone agreed with their theories on specificity and that there was no supporting statistical proof. To try to correct this French, Alexander and George H. Pollock[3] gathered together a group of analysts, physicians and statisticians and carried out a courageous and painstaking piece of research. Their line of thought was that if certain psychosomatic diseases were brought about by specific psychodynamic factors, then presentation of carefully collected analytical observations, on patients with known psychosomatic diseases to a panel of trained analysts, should enable them to make a correct diagnosis on the basis of the specificity of these observations. Patients suffering from seven distinct psychosomatic diseases were interviewed individually by an analyst and the proceedings were tape recorded. These records were then processed to exclude all references or hints about the nature of the medical diagnosis. Each report was submitted to a panel of analytical judges for a decision on the appropriate diagnosis. As a check the same reports were studied by physicians without analytical knowledge, but not biased one way or another on the subject. They too were called upon to make a diagnosis which they did on a basis mainly of general medical reasoning. The difference in the success rate between analytical and medical assessment would again confirm the value of a knowledge of the specific psychodynamic pattern associated with each disease. In the event a total of eighty-three patients of mixed sexes were studied. The analytical judges scored a fifty per cent success rate, the physicians scored a twenty-five per cent success rate and this compared with fourteen per cent (ie one in seven) which could have been guessed by chance. These figures are not clear cut to us although statistically they would be accepted as being better than would be expected by chance. So on their own assessment this group could only provide limited support for their theory of psychosomatic specificity. How do other workers regard this theory?

In general it can be said that the theory is less acceptable as time passes and more knowledge about the psychosomatic diseases comes to light. There is a strong hereditary and constitutional element in these diseases and as this becomes clearer the validity of the specific psychodynamic role recedes. In a chapter on childhood asthma in *Modern Trends in Psychosomatic Medicine* Phillip Pinkerton and Corrina M. Weaver[4] have this to say.

> These studies (referring to specific psychoanalytical formulations) forfeit their claim to validity through failure to acknowledge the somatic substrate [underlying physical condition] which is fundamental to our understanding of the asthmatic state. Manifestly no analytical construct can ever be said to produce the asthmatic's labile bronchus, yet by emphasizing ambivalence and early childhood experience as factors influencing the course of the illness – the way the labile bronchus behaves – psychoanalytical theory does tie in with data from other disciplines and, therefore, does retain some relevance though not in a causal sense.

Similar interpretations could be usefully applied to the psychological aspects of other psychosomatic disorders.

Another analytical concept is that of secondary gain. The patient may suffer intense physical discomfort, and on rare occasions even lose his life, as for example in a severe attack of asthma, but nevertheless it is claimed there is a psychological gain. Some part of his mind is considered to be protected. Richard W. Garnett[5] put it like this, 'A person may find it useful or necessary, or he may prefer to be sick.' He described the case of a young woman who started having attacks of asthma on taking up her first job. She promptly left the job and lived at home with her parents. To her, asthma was an excuse for avoiding employment or marriage. Robert D. Gillespie[6] expressed similar views. Asthma to him was often a protection or a mode of escape from an intolerable situation. Few asthmatics would agree with these ideas.

A conscious and agonizing choice between life and death has sometimes to be made. Martyrs have died at the stake rather than betray an ideal. It would be too grotesque a proposition that the asthmatic makes a conscious choice between an attack, with its attendant dangers, and submission to some hurtful psychological experience. In any case how can he bring on an attack? A depressed and hysterical person may injure himself to escape feelings of guilt or an unwelcome situation, and he can readily find an instrument with which to hurt himself. But can the asthmatic turn on the tap at will? There is some evidence that a modified, partial attack is possible as a consequence of fear or a conditioned reflex. It has often been observed that an attack can be brought about by the sight of an artificial flower to which the asthmatic is sensitive. It will bring on an immediate attack probably through spasms of bronchial muscles as a result of overactivity of the autonomic nervous system. Some psychiatrists have also suggested that a voluntary forced expiration can produce an inward distortion of the soft posterior wall of bronchi and so cause narrowing of the passage and wheezing. A healthy subject can indeed do this if he tries but it would not be called asthma. No, the true asthmatic attack is brought about by three major changes in the bronchial tubes. The circular muscle around the tube goes into spasm, the lining of the tube is thickened by congestion and allergic inflammation and the cavity of the tube is filled with an allergic exudate resembling a jelly-like liquid. Psychological factors may bring on an immediate attack by spasm of muscle but it is difficult to believe that the full blown attack which must include the other two changes referred to can take place on this basis. If we rule out conscious choice we are then told it is subconscious. Subconscious processes may be involved, but once this is accepted the words choice, gain and escape begin to lose their meaning. Surely the more sensible, and more generous, approach would be to reject the concept of secondary gain and to talk instead of the patient paying a penalty for a mistaken attitude, whether conscious or subconscious, by developing asthma. For example, we have seen an asthmatic reject help by reason of false pride and a need to express independence and as a result suffer from loneliness and resentment which led later to asthma. This is a delayed response and is mediated by accepted mechanisms including infective, allergic and hormonal processes. Maybe the whole problem is a semantic one. Is the patient escaping into asthma or is he paying the penalty of lack of insight and wisdom? In our view it is the latter. Escape into asthma is a sick way of describing the situation; it is like talking of the benefits of jumping out of the frying pan into the fire. No one escapes that way. We would like to see far less use of the words 'gain' and 'escape' when referring to the asthmatic. All their efforts are directed to living as normal a life as possible. Perhaps their mistakes bring about suffering, but such is the case with us all. On rare occasion an asthmatic attack might be utilized to gain sympathy or escape from a situation, but in our view the attack is already there and is just exaggerated for the occasion. We are always surprised by the reverse situation, by the courage and persistence of most patients in their attempts to carry on with their normal duties. Take, for example, the asthmatic schoolboy who struggles to get to school and bravely plays games in spite of his handicap, unlike other children who relish an opportunity to play truant.

Our conclusion is that a specific psychodynamic picture cannot be regarded as causal in psychosomatic disease, but that in a proportion of cases it may play a part. This does not imply that we have a clear picture of a specific psychodynamic pattern for each disease. Analysts would not even agree amongst themselves about this. Freudians would dispute with Jungians and Jungians with Adlerians. We have also considerable hesitation in accepting the orthodox analytic view of the psychodynamic process. We do not want to side-track the issue by talking at length on analytical formulations, but briefly we must say that in these formulations of how a person develops an inner conflict and a vulnerable and unadaptable personality, there seems to be far too great an emphasis on sexuality between parent and child and far too great a link between such matters as anal and oral function and higher mental processes. Perhaps as analysts pay greater attention to other instinctual drives the emphasis on the sexual and erotic will lessen and a meeting point will be established between analysts, orthodox psychiatrists and physicians. In the meantime we can agree that some diseases have a large content of psychological trauma and tension and that almost all diseases are in some way influenced by psychological processes.

Few diseases exemplify psychosomatic concepts better than thyrotoxicosis. In this condition the thyroid gland becomes overactive and produces an excess of the hormone Thyroxine, which regulates the rate of general activity of the body. The patient, who is usually a woman, develops a swelling in the neck, protrusion of the eyes, a racing pulse and an anxious, excitable behaviour. Her raised metabolic rate is accompanied by weight loss and the outstretched fingers show a fine tremor. The exact nature of this common condition is unknown, but there are both mental and physical factors in its development and these appear to be necessary and complementary. The psychological element was seen to be one of a patient suddenly thrust into a world of excessive responsibility, through loss of a parent or parent figure, on whom she was overdependent. By reason of immaturity she is unable to cope and reacts excessively to the stressful situation. Her dreams are threatening and often have a content of funeral processions and coffins. This early picture, arising out of a psychoanalytic approach, is perhaps overdramatic and a less extreme and less specific picture now tends to be painted. Although there may be loss of a parent or parent figure, we find more commonly a situation in which an unprepared person is called upon to face a considerable increase in responsibility. For example, a woman of thirty-five, who was coping quite well with a family which included an asthmatic and eczematous boy, developed thyrotoxicosis when her husband fell ill with a serious but transient illness. The psychological component of the disease is now widely accepted, yet psychotherapy is not the first line of treatment. Specific antithyroid drugs or surgery are required in most cases. In milder cases, not requiring physical treatment, and in cases which have gone into a remission as a result of successful medical treatment, limited psychotherapy of a supportive kind and perhaps advice urging a temporary shedding of excess responsibility are of help.

The physical element of thyrotoxicosis is not fully understood, but there is evidence from animal experiment that the adrenal cortex is not as active as it should be.

An attractive theory which would bring together the mental and physical factors in the origin of the disease would be as follows:– Illness or death of a member of the family places excessive demands on the patient. At first there is a physiological overactivity of the thyroid gland in response to stress. After a period of continuous anxiety, coupled, perhaps, with insomnia, chronic fatigue, associated with an insufficient output of cortisol, sets in and antibodies are allowed to form to a special part of the envelope of the thyroid cell which stimulates the cell to prolonged and pathological overactivity. (This state of fatigue is a most interesting condition and will be fully discussed later in the book, as will the formation of antibodies in auto-immune disease.)

Rheumatoid arthritis is also widely regarded as a psychosomatic disease and if we can substantiate this claim then our approach to prevention and treatment will be radically altered. In 1950 the Empire Rheumatism Council boldly declared on the basis of a questionnaire of patients suffering from Rheumatoid Arthritis, that there was no evidence for the participation of any special psychological or emotional trauma in the development of the disease. Many physicians and psychiatrists have differed with this conclusion and continue to differ. In 1936, Phillip Ellman and S. D. Mitchell[7] noticed the frequency of worry, pressure of work, marital disharmony and similar factors in the period preceding the onset of the disease. This study was not statistically significant because comparison had not been made with a control group, ie a group not suffering from Rheumatoid Arthritis. But many other controlled studies pointed to the same situation. Alexander,[8] giving an analytical assessment, considered that the sufferer, usually a woman, finds it difficult to handle her aggressive, hostile impulses. Her solution is by self-control and benevolent tyranny over others. The typical mother of the arthritic would be restrictive and the child would react by excessive physical and tomboy activity. Arthritis might develop when hostile impulses are blocked by some change in the life situation. For example, loss of a person whom the patient previously dominated was a common precipitating condition. He also felt that 'the arthritic process is unfavourably influenced by the increased muscle tonus that results from simultaneous mobilization of aggressive impulses and their inhibition – a kind of straight-jacket situation.'

More recent work in this field takes a broader view; observer error is lessened by modern psychological techniques and by using more than one assessor. Rudolf Moos and George Solomon[9] carried out a careful comparison of the personality and behaviour of arthritic women with their nearest non-affected sister. In these circumstances parental influence and early domestic environment would be similar. Various personality traits and attitudes were assessed as objectively as possible using accepted psychological scales and techniques. Whereas siblings (unaffected sisters) regarded their mothers as benevolent and good parents, the patients were more critical and often thought of them as intolerant, strict and lacking in affection. Fathers were also considered by the patients to be less perfect. Whereas siblings looked upon their marriages as reasonably happy, the patients either approved whole-heartedly of their husbands or disapproved of them but put up with them. Siblings would express their feelings openly to their husbands and sometimes quarrel with them, whilst patients tolerated them and never quarrelled with them. Contrary to the findings of previous workers both patients and controls were highly independent. Patients were less able to express their hostility, were more conscious of their duties and responsibilities and were more likely to sacrifice their own interests.

As to the life situation at the onset of the disease Moos and Solomon found that chronic, long-term stress was more often responsible than simple discrete or short-term stress. This is in keeping with the Cluster Theory of disease and also with the concept of chronic fatigue.

They carried out another most interesting piece of research on healthy relatives of patients with rheumatoid arthritis. In a group of relatives they found twenty-one who had a rheumatoid factor (a specific auto-antibody) in the blood. These were compared with a similar number without this factor. The presence of the factor indicates a greater predisposition to the disease. Were there any psychological mechanisms which had protected these susceptible people from the disease? Detailed comparison showed that the women with a rheumatoid factor, but no apparent disease, tended to have well functioning defences and be psychiatrically relatively symptom free. Those without a rheumatoid factor had a more vulnerable personality and suffered more from a host of neurotic symptoms. It seemed then, that in order to remain healthy, the relatives with a positive rheumatoid factor had to have a stable personality and had to be capable of coping and adapting.

In conclusion then we may say that persons with a genetic or constitutional predisposition to rheumatoid arthritis may develop the disease if subjected to considerable emotional conflict and if their psychological defence mechanisms are weak. If the reverse is true then in spite of a constitutional tendency, the disease would not develop.

Here again the original analytical formulation appears to be too specific and rigid, while, nevertheless, there is evidence of excessive vulnerability in these patients. Their high sense of duty and concern for others leads them to accept responsibilities and carry out tasks in excess of their strength.

If we accept the basic tenet of Psychosomatic Medicine that psychological trauma plays an important role in the origin and maintenance of some diseases and a lesser role in almost all diseases we should begin to ask the question: who should treat the patient's psychological problems? Should it be the General Practitioner, the

Consultant Physician, the General Psychiatrist, the Analytically orientated Psychiatrist or a new breed of specialist the Consultant Psychosomatic Physician if such a specialist existed? The answer is not as complex as it might be. General Practitioners are well aware of psychological and social problems and most of them find it easy to establish sympathetic and friendly contact with their patients. There is increasing emphasis on psychiatry and psychotherapy in the training of undergraduates and postgraduates and the psychiatric content of psychosomatic illness is more widely appreciated and understood. So the family physician should, and would wish to, take an interest in the less dramatic forms of psychosomatic disease and be able to treat the patient in respect to both mental and physical aspects of his illness and help him, perhaps aided by social workers, with his social and family problems. The great advantage of this system is that mental and physical treatments are co-ordinated and there is less chance of one or the other therapy being forgotten. His one great problem is lack of time and this is something the Government and the profession should rectify. There is too great a gap between ideal treatment and practical treatment. The detailed history – biographical, social and psychological – which is needed and the subsequent psychotherapy, however basic and simple, require more than an average GP consultation time of five or seven minutes. Once we accept the importance of psychological factors in disease our concept of Doctor-Patient interviews will have to change radically.

If the illness is more complex or severe, then a hospital consultation or admission will be needed and here again we would expect the physician or surgeon to be able to deal with both the psychiatric and physical aspects of most of the psychosomatic diseases. In this he will have the help of his junior colleagues and social workers. Again a plea has to be made to give the Hospital Consultant sufficient time to talk to the patient in an unhurried and relaxed fashion. The rushed outpatient consultation and the limited bedside contact which prevail at present are not conducive to good psychosomatic treatment. When one considers the full gravity of a condition such as active rheumatoid arthritis and its possibly devastating effect on the life of the patient, or, for that matter, the gravity of some of the other psychosomatic diseases such as ulcerative colitis, asthma or high blood pressure, we have a right to expect that the Health Service will not only ensure adequate physical treatment of patients but also, as far as is humanly possible, deal fully and competently with their psychological and social problems.

There will be special cases when a psychiatrist should be called in either where the physician is not psychiatrically orientated, or where the patient has more serious psychiatric disorders, such as a deep depression or psychotic symptoms. The psychiatrist should preferably be interested in psychosomatic problems and not be so occupied with his purely psychiatric and administrative work that he cannot find the time to deal with psychiatric aspects of predominantly physical disease.

Should one enlist the services of an analyst? This is a difficult problem and is partly solved by two factors. Firstly, analysis is extremely costly and time-consuming and is barely available in the setting of the NHS. Secondly, a number of analysts would not be sufficiently interested in psychosomatic medicine nor be sufficiently trained in the biological aspects of medicine. We must also bear in mind the lack of statistical evidence for therapeutic success in this field. John F. O'Connor,[10] in an article entitled 'A comprehensive approach to the treatment of ulcerative colitis' discusses the role of psychotherapy in a series of nine hundred patients whose cases were reviewed retrospectively. Only 104 of these had been seen by a psychiatrist; and only fifty-seven of these were followed for a long enough period to be assessed, thirty-eight were treated by psycho-analytically orientated psychotherapy. Of these thirteen received brief therapy (less than twenty sessions), while six had over four hundred hours of analysis each. So that even in the United States of America, where this work took place, of nine hundred cases of ulcerative colitis only six had extensive analytical therapy. No statistical evidence can be based on such small groups.

The fifty-seven cases mentioned above who had had some psychotherapy, were matched with fifty-seven control patients and a comparison of progress over several years was made, based on the severity of symptoms and the appearance of the lining of the gut. There was a slight but definite overall advantage in favour of the group treated by psychotherapy.

We must leave this matter unresolved. If the family physician, the hospital consultant, or patient for that matter, wish to organize psychotherapy on an analytical basis and if the necessary opportunity and finance exist, then, provided the analyst is interested in that particular psychosomatic problem, there is no reason why it should not be undertaken.

There will also be the more conventional psychiatrist who has had analytical training or experience, and he may wish to give a shortened form of psychotherapy suited to the needs of the patient.

We do not think it matters particularly which form of psychotherapy a patient receives so long as it is given with sincerity, knowledge and concern. A meeting on this subject at a chest clinic illustrates this point. A medically qualified hypnotist, a psychiatrist interested in psychosomatic medicine and an analyst all talked about their techniques and results in the treatment of asthma. Their achievements appeared to be very similar. Perhaps we are all good with the special tools which we have learnt to use. Rice can be eaten effectively with forks, spoons or chopsticks.

Perhaps a new specialty of psychosomatic medicine will develop in time in this country. It is not too far fetched a concept as the diseases which are at present acknowledged as being psychosomatic cause a great deal of invalidism and loss of working time. Moreover the list of psychosomatic diseases is expanding. The proposed specialist would be required to have an extensive training both in medicine and psychiatry and have a special multifactorial approach based on this knowledge. For the time being we would be happy if family doctors, hospital physicians and psychiatrists were to be given the opportunity of treating their patients affected by this group of diseases, with all the care they need, as whole human beings on the understanding that the psyche and soma cannot be split.

We have still a lot to discuss in the field of psychosomatic medicine and perhaps it would be better to continue this subject later in the book when dealing with social and work stress.

6

*

The Cluster Theory of Disease

UP TO THE TIME when Thomas Holmes[1] and Richard Rahe[2] produced their classical work on the cluster theory of illness there had been much speculation on the relationship between misfortune and stressful experience on the one hand and illness on the other. Then, following a simple but brilliant piece of research, there arose an appreciation that these events were related to the point of mathematical certitude.

The success of their approach depended upon a satisfactory mathematical grading of stressful experience. All of us experience suffering or change in our life situation; but how does one compare the experience of one person with that of another in order to determine who has suffered most? The answer was unexpected but effective. It was to question the man in the street, or rather lots of men and women in the street. A list of some forty significant experiences, which any of us might undergo, was compiled and submitted to a large number of people who were asked to give each a numerical value, according to the gravity of the experience and the effort needed to adapt to it. The most stressful experience would be rated at one hundred units while a non-stressful experience would be rated at zero units. Examples might be – loss of wife, husband or child: one hundred units; loss of job: sixty units; large bank overdraft: thirty units; small overdraft: twenty units; and so on. Pleasurable events which require effort or adaptation were also given a score, and so promotion or marriage of a son or daughter might rank as ten units. The rating scale was based on the average of a large number of valuations of each event and the units were called Life Change Units (LCUs).

TABLE I

Results of Social Readjustment Rating Questionnaire

	Life Event	*Mean Value*		*Life Event*	*Mean Value*
1	Death of spouse	100	22	Change in responsibilities at work	29
2	Divorce	73	23	Son or daughter leaving home	29
3	Marital separation	65	24	Trouble with in-laws	29
4	Jail term	63	25	Outstanding personal achievement	28
5	Death of close family member	63	26	Wife begins or stops work	26
6	Personal injury or illness	53	27	Begin or end school	26
7	Marriage	50	28	Change in living conditions	25
8	Fired at work	47	29	Revision of personal habits	24
9	Marital reconciliation	45	30	Trouble with boss	23
10	Retirement	45	31	Change in work hours or conditions	20
11	Change in health of family member	44	32	Change in residence	20
12	Pregnancy	40	33	Change in schools	20
13	Sexual difficulties	39	34	Change in recreation	19
14	Gain of new family member	39	35	Change in church activities	19
15	Business readjustment	39	36	Change in social activities	18
16	Change in financial state	38	37	Mortgage or loan less than $10,000	17
17	Death of close friend	37	38	Change in sleeping habits	16
18	Change to different line of work	36	39	Change in number of family get-togethers	15
19	Change in number of arguments with spouse	35	40	Change in eating habits	13
20	Mortgage over $10,000	31	41	Vacation	13
21	Foreclosure of mortgage or loan	30	42	Minor violations of the law	11

Taken from Rahe, R. H. (1969), in *Psychotropic Drug Response. Advances in Prediction*, May, P. R. A., and Wittenborn, J. R., Illinois, p. 97.

The standard questionnaire containing a list of experiences was called the Schedule of Recent Experiences. By completing such a schedule for a given period, perhaps the preceding six or twelve months, or two years, a mathematically valid figure could be given to the patient's stressful experiences over that period.

The next problem was to find a group of subjects or a population which could be observed and assessed for a sufficiently long period of time. Since the research workers in point were naval medical officers, this presented no difficulty. The project was carried out with the help of US naval personnel aboard three cruisers. This provided an admirable setting for the experiment, involving a co-operative group of men, whose medical status could be meticulously followed over the whole period of their tour of duty. After careful briefing LCUs were recorded for successive six month periods over the two years preceding the tour. It was later found that the final six month period was most relevant and this was used in the eventual analysis.

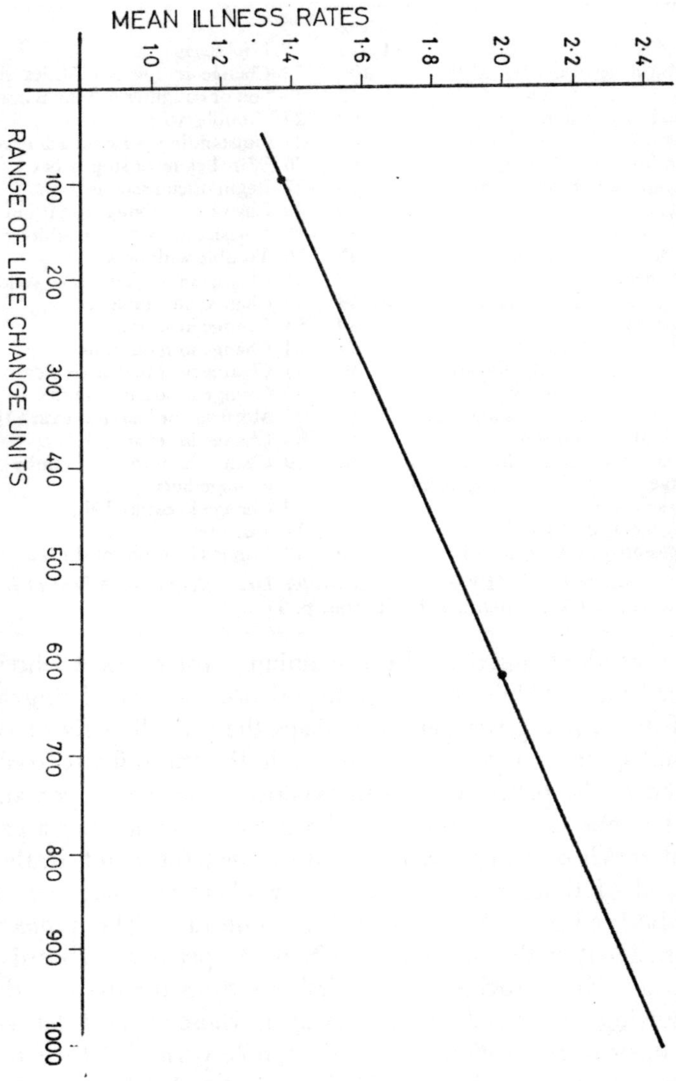

Fig VI. Diagram to show correlation between life change units and mean illness rates

The degree of co-operation on the part of the men was remarkable. Some ninety-five per cent of the 2,664 men took part. Each visit to the medical clinic was noted and at the end of the tour of duty Mean Illness Rates (MIRs) were calculated on the basis of men's sickness attendances. A statistical correlation was found between the MIRs and the range of LCUs. At the lower end of the scale one hundred LCUs were associated with 1.4 MIRs, while at the top end of the scale six hundred LCUs were coupled with two MIRs (see Fig. VI).

These results, covering such a large group of men, were statistically significant and proved beyond doubt, for the first time, that, the more stressful life experiences are crowded together, the more illness results; that a cluster of significant life changes will be followed by a cluster of diseases. It might be objected that the sample of subjects in the research (entirely healthy males) was not representative, but similar research among mixed civilian populations has confirmed the findings.

The corollary of this must be that in the prevention of disease, we should take into account the social environment and consider how pressures on the individual can be lessened, for they have at last been shown to be among the silent villains of the piece.

The next matter of interest was to see whether the severity of stressful experience is related to the severity of disease. This proposition was studied by Rahe, Joseph McKean and Arthur,[3] in a group of retired Service personnel most of whom were on a one hundred per cent disability pension for neurotic or psychotic illness.

They graded the severity of an illness by assessing the risk of death or serious disability which could be attached to it. So in a grade one illness, ie one of minor severity, the risk would be less than one in ten thousand, while in a grade five illness, ie one of considerable severity, the risk would be less than one in ten.

As these men had been in the services for long periods of time, their illnesses could be traced from records for ten to twenty years and LCUs could be correlated with both frequency and severity of illness. The mean yearly LCU rating was found to be seventy-two. The mean of LCUs prior to a cluster of minor severity (grades one to two) was 130 and prior to a cluster of high severity (grades three, four and five) was 164.

It is instructive to pick out a diagram of LCUs and illness over

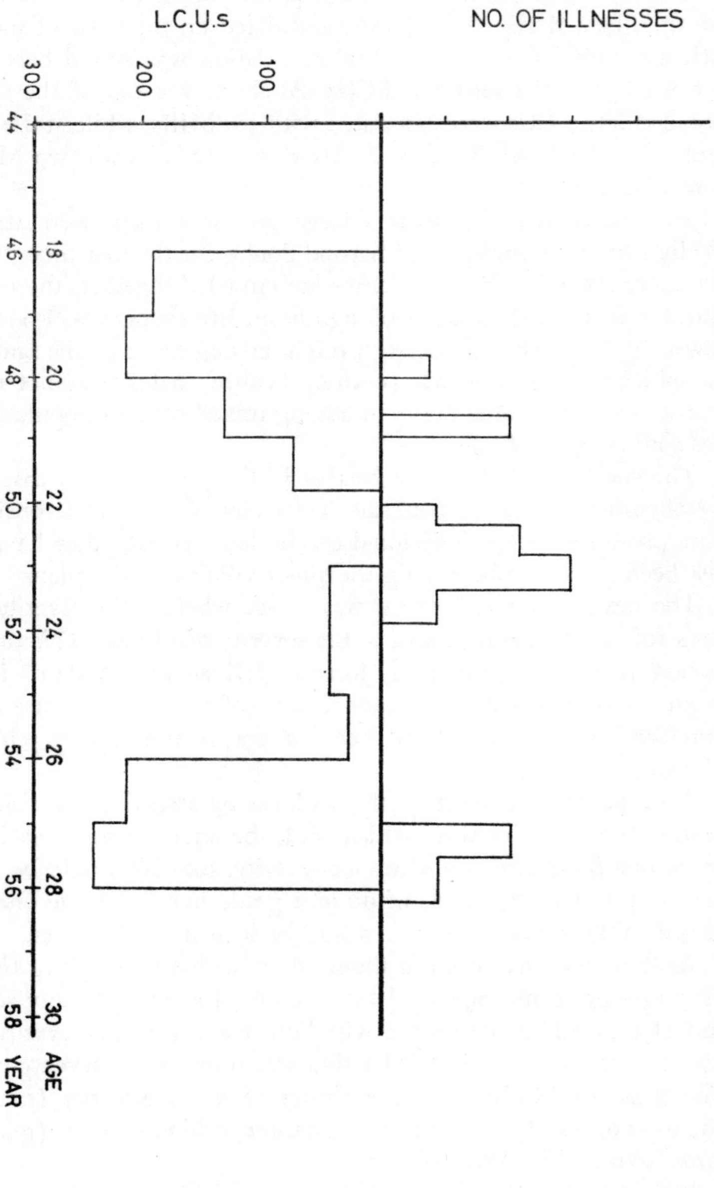

Fig VII. Diagram showing 'icebergs' of life change units followed by 'peaks' of illnesses

a period of years from a selected case history. We will see clusters of LCUs looking like icebergs followed by clusters of illness like small mountain peaks. The diagram (Fig. VII) gives us an idea. If only we could abolish the icebergs we might thereby remove the following peaks. This, of course, is over-ambitious and totally impractical. But what may perhaps be possible is to counteract the effect of the iceberg by precautionary measures – perhaps increased rest, psychotherapy or appropriate drugs.

It may be that our ancestors had a better understanding of the connection between bereavement and illness, for they observed a long period of mourning after the death of a loved relative. They must have sensed that withdrawal from active life at such times, was psychologically useful and allowed the wounded mind to heal. We might consider a therapeutic holiday after being sacked from a job or after financial disaster.

Similar work was carried out by Allen Wyler, Minoru Masuda and Holmes.[4] They used a Seriousness of Illness Rating scale (SIRs) in which forty-two disease items were graded according to their degree of severity. 232 patients were reviewed and asked to complete a Schedule of Recent Experiences for periods of six months, one year and two years. The researchers found a significant correlation between the LCU score in all periods and the SIRs. The greater the LCU score the more serious the cluster of illness which followed, and this was particularly so in relation to chronic disease.

We begin to see a link between the Psychosomatic diseases, which are in the main chronic (witness asthma, high blood pressure, peptic ulcer, rheumatoid arthritis, and so on) and preceding non-specific stressful events.

So far we have been dealing with LUCs over long periods, say, six months to two years, and significant illnesses. But what about day-to-day experiences and problems in relation to minor illness? Are they too connected? Thomas S. Holmes and Thomas H. Holmes,[5] in 1970, wrote an article humorously entitled 'Short term Intrusions into the Life Style Routine'. College students (obviously changed into professional hypochondriacs for a time) were asked to keep a Schedule of Daily Experiences (SDE) and also a day-to-day list of their minor symptoms and illnesses. Not surprisingly the outcome of this experiment was that the incidence of minor complaints was correlated with the pressures and problems weighing on them. At first glance this research seems trivial, but when we look at it more carefully it throws some light on previously mysterious events. We are all aware of minor ailments, such as headaches, twinges of joint pain and catarrh which seem to come without good cause. Now we can partly blame the day to day strains of life. But more important, we begin to understand the mechanism of such periodic conditions as 'week end' migraine and asthma. The work of Holmes and Holmes seems to confirm our impression that the hectic activity of the working week with its problems and increasing fatigue tends to lead to these troubles.

And, so, in the last few years we have had proved to us by statistical methods what the more observant have always felt to be true – that the crowding together of human experiences, both unpleasant and pleasant, will result in an incidence of illness above the average; that the greater the drama and unpleasantness of these experiences, the more serious the illness is likely to be, particularly when it is chronic illness. Minor illnesses are not exempt from this logic and they too tend to follow our daily minor stresses. The adaptive machinery is called into play by these life changes. Each adaptation uses up certain resources. If the system is over-taxed the resources fail and maladaptation takes place with consequent illness.

7

*

Fatigue: An Exploration

TRAUMATIC EXPERIENCES IN LIFE may lead, as we have seen, to ill health. Yet not everyone is equally susceptible and the robust and adaptable seem to escape the penalties paid by the weaker. Is there any means of telling who will succumb and who will not? In certain diseases such as diabetes and cancer, screening procedures will help to detect the early case. Chronic fatigue which appears to afflict the less robust and possibly less adaptable members of the community could be considered to be an early warning signal and herald the development of a wide group of rheumatic and allergic disorders. This chapter will be more speculative and less conformist than its predecessors. Cast iron statistical proof will not be produced, but compensation for this deficiency will be made by the introduction of a new outlook which will help our understanding of some common diseases and perhaps their prevention.

We are sometimes confronted by words or ideas so nebulous and indistinct that we fight shy of trying to understand them and turn them to our service. Such a word is 'fatigue'. It is used again and again in ordinary conversation. It describes how we feel after a gruelling experience or at the end of a tough day. It means something to the person who complains and to the friend who sympathizes. But to the scientific mind it remains, in spite of a little understanding here and there, a blank, enigmatic, indefinable thing. The subject of fatigue has been under consideration at several international conferences (for example the Third International Congress on Psychosomatic Medicine held in Paris in 1966, was devoted entirely to this subject) but little that is constructive or informative has emerged. The Conferences start with a puzzle and finish with a mystery, with the result that the dispirited participants shelve the enigmatic condition for a few more years.

Physiologists, by definition, are concerned with normal functioning of cells, tissues and organs. Dr Albert Hemingway in 1952,[1] put the physiologist's understanding of fatigue like this 'Fatigue is a decrement [decrease] in output with continued use of tissue or organ, the process being reversible and recovery taking place during rest.' Although excessive work or a hostile environment may result in a pathological process and ill health, it is not the task of the physiologist to follow the process to the stage of disease. One would scarcely expect him to look at fatigue as a forerunner of illness and this is indeed so. The biochemical changes in muscle fatigue are complex, but we need not study them here as we are not really concerned with reversible muscle fatigue but rather with a more general type of fatigue, in which the brain and some endocrine glands are probably implicated. Physiologists do not appear to consider that fatigue is related to the pituitary-adrenal axis in spite of the work of Selye, who implies this very strongly when he describes the stage of exhaustion in his discussion of the General Adaptation Syndrome.

Fatigue in Industry has special implications. The objectives of Health workers in this field are twofold. Firstly, there is the safety and wellbeing of the worker, and secondly, the boosting of output to its maximum. Fortunately, these aims are to a large extent, complementary. Fatigue is inimical to both, and it should be possible to decrease this unwanted state by manipulating the environment and introducing adequate rest periods. It was shown many years ago that a shortening of working hours and the introduction of appropriate breaks from work resulted in increased output, and that the avoidance of fatigue decreased the incidence of industrial accidents. Wise management accordingly takes the necessary measures, with benefit to their own profits and the wellbeing of the workers.

Shiftwork is a potent cause of fatigue in Industry by running counter to man's natural rhythm of work and sleep. In chapter two we described the circadian output of the Adrenocorticotrophic hormone (ACTH). The body possesses a remarkably accurate internal clock which ensures that sufficient ACTH is produced in the early hours of the morning so that there should be in turn, an ample supply of cortisol on waking to help meet daytime demands of work and stress. As night approaches the supply of ACTH and cortisol is allowed to fall. In a similar fashion there are many other circadian rhythms geared to the body's needs at various times of the day and night. For example adrenaline output is highest between 8.00 am and 8.00 pm and reaches its lowest point at 2.00 am. Liver stores of glycogen, the precursor of glucose, are lowest after midnight. When, therefore, a man is asked to work at night he is working at a time when his body is totally unprepared both psychologically and physically, and fatigue, inefficiency and error supervene. If he persists in the unnatural attempt the internal clock is slowly reset to coincide with the work clock but this adjustment may take a week or more. As night shifts are socially less attractive than day shifts both managers and workers attempt to distribute this unpopular shift between the work force and the worst possible compromise is made of the rotating night shift. No sooner has the internal clock adjusted when the man changes his shift and the clock is asked to go into reverse, taking many further days to readjust. It seems logical therefore to continue a night shift, once it has been instituted, for some months so as to avoid frequent disruption of the circadian rhythm and consequent fatigue.

Many factors are thought to enter into the development of Industrial fatigue, some being well substantiated while others are purely speculative. For example, morale and choice play an important role. Where group morale is high and where the worker participates in his work by choice, there are fewer complaints of fatigue. Where the worker participates unwillingly, morale is low and fatigue is readily experienced and made an excuse for slowing down. Some psychiatrists talk of 'managerial fatigue' which is ignored by the sufferer who spurs himself on to further achievement and 'worker fatigue', which allows escape from an imposed and resented task. One can be sure that all managers are not so noble nor workers so unco-operative.

Some observers divide fatigue into true, organic fatigue and neurotic fatigue. The latter is thought to stem from an inability to sublimate aggressive drives into work. Aggression then finds an outlet in the passive reaction of fatigue.

One could elaborate on the psychological aspects of Industrial fatigue and argue for or against certain concepts, but however important these psychological problems are, they are less pressing than the main issue, which is whether Industrial fatigue is a major cause of serious and widespread ill health, or whether it has only a marginal influence.

Certain conditions in industry have long been known to give rise to specific diseases, for example silicosis, due to inhalation of mineral particles, cancer of the bladder by reason of carcinogenic chemicals and various allergies of skin and lungs; and these conditions are being prevented by legally enforcible measures of hygiene, but stress resulting from the industrial environment has not, until recently, been regarded as a serious factor in disease provocation. Few would have regarded heart disease or the rheumatic complaints as being the consequence of industrial stress. Now these possibilities are the subject of intense research in stress laboratories and evidence is accumulating that social and industrial conditions play their part in the development of illness. Indeed it would be strange if illness could result only from factors behind the front door of one's home. A large part of our lives is spent in the setting of factory or office and, as described in chapter 12, we must, in future, take these work factors into account.

One of the outstanding students of fatigue in the broader field of Medicine and Psychiatry is Samuel H. Bartley, whose book, *Fatigue, Mechanism and Management* was published in 1965.[2] He described fatigue as a 'sensory cognitive syndrome which includes tiredness, aversion to work, body discomfort, ineffectiveness in performance . . . a self felt assessment of inadequacy . . . and the experience of futility . . . with the desire to escape'. This is an excellent description of the state of fatigue. Bartley went on:

> to summarize, it may be said that instead of using fatigue as a single or loose catch all term, we had better recognize the involvement of a group of quite distinguishable elements in the total situation. They are impairment, disorganization, discomfort largely localized in muscles, work decrement, and finally fatigue. . . . Impairment is the reduced ability of the cells to function. Disorganization is modification in the ways of cells, tissues and organs working together. . . . Discomfort arises through sensory mechanisms being affected by tissue changes including those called impairment. Work decrement is the measurable drop in activity of muscles measured in energistic terms or the drop in intellectual productivity measured in other terms. . . . Fatigue is the individual's assessment of his condition with reference to his immediate task. . . .

All this is beautifully descriptive, but it puts forward no suggestion as to the mechanisms involved.

Bartley made a useful distinction between immediate or acute fatigue and chronic fatigue. He considered that situations which may give rise to acute fatigue are – a high level of energy expenditure, prolonged activity, and conditions in the environment that limit activity such as excessive humidity or extremes of temperature. There are also psychological situations predisposing to fatigue such as elements tending to frustrate performance, demands too exacting for the capacity of a specific body mechanism and activity in the face of goals which are too remote.

On the other hand Bartley writes: 'Chronic fatigue may be looked upon from the standpoint of some deficiency in the individual in question.' Yes, but what deficiency? Bartley hazards no guess.

Bartley has most ably defined fatigue and given us an intelligent breakdown into its component parts, some of which are measurable. Physiologists can measure muscle fatigue and fatigue of the nerve supplying the muscle. Fatigue of an organ can be roughly assessed by various means such as measurement of output or by chemical and staining techniques. For example, the fatigued adrenal cortex will show a decrease in its content of ascorbic acid while the fatigued adrenal medulla will show a fainter staining of some of its cells. Intellectual impairment is measurable by psychological tests. It would be more difficult to devise tests for the sensory part of fatigue which is subjective or for the psychological component such as feelings of boredom or inadequacy.

Richard C. Browne, in 1953, made an interesting statement in a paper, 'Fatigue, Fact or Fiction', before a symposium on fatigue under the auspices of the Ergonomics Research Society.[3] He said:

> It is also clearly a fact that performance is related to environment and that it shows a natural diurnal and nocturnal rhythm. But it is a fiction that there is a single entity called fatigue and that the search has only to be long enough to find a single test for it. The human being has many functions and each one fits a different test.

There is little doubt that Browne is right in general and that we will find no single test to cover all aspects of fatigue; but we should not be too pessimistic. If we can pin-point one of the important components of fatigue and measure it, then we shall have achieved a worthwhile result.

In 1966 an annotation in *The Lancet* (12 March) stated plaintively, 'Not much is known about the cause of fatigue even in its simplest form, and one reason is that fatigue is hard to measure.' It goes on to discuss neuro-muscular fatigue and restates physiological knowledge on this subject. In view of the fact that a fatigued muscle will contract again if the strength of the nerve stimulus is increased the writer makes the comment that mental determination or motivation can counteract or delay fatigue.

A distinction is made between muscle fatigue which is rarely disagreeable and may even be pleasant and 'tiredness', which requires stimulation or mental effort to overcome and is thus a central rather than a peripheral state. Tiredness is manifested by decreased performance, inertia, drooping facial muscles and a change in body posture. It is brought on or aggravated by frustration, anxiety and fear.

This distinction between fatigue and tiredness is unconvincing. It would perhaps be better to talk of simple muscular fatigue on the one hand and mental and general fatigue on the other.

The Lancet annotation concludes by asking:

> What is the nature of tiredness at the end of the day's work? Boredom is probably a potent factor, as are perhaps a rising sense of hunger, and the accumulating physical discomfort of circulatory stagnation due to prolonged standing or sitting. Even then, if the work is interesting or rewarding, it is possible to continue for longer than usual without feeling tired.
>
> We are left with some idea of the factors which can make for fatigue, and with the realization that we are ignorant of what really happens in the organism and why certain emotions so powerfully inhibit the will to physical or mental activity. Nor do we know whether tiredness is ever beneficial. It may be a warning, or it may be an escape, according to the individual and the circumstances.

In these last words the interesting suggestion is put forward that fatigue may, in part, be a warning – a signal urging the individual to slow down or rest. This is the theme that we would like to develop later on. But in general *The Lancet* analysis takes us no further than the work of Bartley.

William B. Spaulding in an article 'The Clinical Analysis of Fatigue'[4] gave a physician's point of view. He found that fatigue was the fifth commonest presenting symptom in a series of 4,000 consecutive patients attending a hospital medical clinic, and that it accounted for seven per cent of the total number of patients. (One must remember that many others would admit to fatigue as a secondary symptom on questioning, and the incidence must be much higher than seven per cent.) Indeed, in a series of 450 hospital patients seen by one of us (A.P.), one in five admitted to fatigue either as a primary or a secondary symptom. Spaulding seeks to account for fatigue by simply listing his main physical or psychiatric diagnoses. A psychiatric disorder was to blame in fifty per cent, endocrine or hormonal conditions in nine per cent, blood disorders in seven per cent, carcinoma in three per cent, and so on. The assumption is that fatigue was brought about by the listed disorder, while it is possible that, in a proportion of the cases, the reverse is true and the disorder might have developed as a result of fatigue. In other words, Spaulding takes the conventional view that fatigue is not an entity in its own right, but is always a symptom of pre-existing disease.

M. E. Groover[5] was more imaginative. He described fourteen cases of 'An unusual syndrome responding to Prolonged ACTH therapy'. The main features were depression and a low threshold of fatiguability. Other symptoms were – darkness around the eyes, increased sweating, headache, joint pains, blueness of the nail beds and a greyish tinge to the skin. His laboratory findings included a low Basal Metabolic Rate (BMR) or turnover of body processes, low fasting blood sugar levels and a low output of some steroids in the urine in half the cases. Most of Groover's patients had suffered an influenza-like illness and had been subjected to emotional tension. A prolonged, but limited, course of ACTH in low dosage corrected the symptoms and brought about a rise in the BMR. Groover seems to have hit upon a small group of patients, suffering from post-influenzal fatigue, in whom there was evidence of decreased pituitary-adrenal activity. They would probably have recovered spontaneously and few physicians would nowadays be prompted to give ACTH on these indications. Nevertheless this work is remarkable for being almost the only study which links fatigue, in certain individuals, with relative steroid insufficiency and attempts a plausible explanation of fatigue in scientific terms.

Another approach to fatigue is exemplified in the work of Harvey E. Nüssbaum,[6] and Guilleman. These authors list all the possible causes of fatigue and devise a remedy for each one. The label of chronic fatigue should not really apply to all these patients. True, they suffer from fatigue, but this is simply of a secondary nature and it is the primary cause which requires treatment. Patients suffering from the many forms of anaemia, thyroid deficiency, protein or vitamin deficiency, depression, and so on, will exhibit fatigue among a host of other symptoms and will recover when specific treatment is given. One of the points Guilleman makes deserves particular attention. He claims that in fatigue due to emotional tension the output of seventeen Ketosteroids (breakdown products of some corticosteroids) in the urine is decreased. This is in keeping with the findings of Groover. Indeed, if we search the literature carefully enough, we find the occasional student of the fatigue state who will stick out his neck and assert that some degree of suprarenal cortical inactivity may be found in that condition. Nüssbaum also makes an interesting and pertinent remark when he states, 'Fatigue without activity is unphysiological.'

Finally we have the psychological approach to fatigue. Held[7] gives a good résumé of the analytical psychiatrist's view. A whole range of emotions and psychological motivations will influence fatigue. Boredom, interest, fear, the impulse to satisfy basic needs and the frustration of these needs and desires all play their part. According to this author there are four basic mechanisms for neurotic fatigue. Firstly, hysterical, which includes reactive fatigue and everything connecting tiredness with emotion. Expressions used by fatigued subjects convey this emotional element, for example 'dead tired' or 'I am tired of'. Secondly, the fatigue of the compulsive neurotic which results from inner conflicts. Thirdly, a masochistic, self-destructive type of fatigue as has already been described when we considered managerial fatigue. This kind of fatigue has certain similarities to addiction, work being like a drug which dulls the senses. Lastly, the fatigue of the psychotic or severely mentally disturbed patient, which may be due to gross mental overactivity and need not be enlarged upon.

When Held considers the psychosomatic manifestations of fatigue, he talks of the tiredness of the subject with a low blood sugar, to be found (so he claims) in boredom and of 'those uprooted from their surroundings who have to manage without the life sustaining stimulus of their hypothalamic-hypophyseal [pituitary] system.' This last concept is valuable, and emphasizes the great importance of interest and motivation in summoning our energies through stimulation of the pituitary-adrenal axis. One can well imagine a fatigued person who will spring into action when the possibility of gratification of some of his cherished needs arises or perhaps an urgent threat to his security. Here again is the realization that one aspect of fatigue is the integrity and activity of the pituitary-adrenal axis.

Held ends his dissertation with a typically poetic analytical passage.

> How far apart are the happiness of intrauterine life and the suckling child from the condition of exhaustion, the tendency of emotional regression, the boredom, the yearnings and the empty existence of the tired modern man. Yet at the same time how close they are when the exhausted individual retreats into sleep, safety and the primitive pursuit of the pleasure principle.

Some workers in Psychosomatic medicine make a distinction between neurotic and psychosomatic fatigue. It is thought that in the former the psychological disturbance is primarily in the cerebral cortex and the hypothalamus is affected secondarily, while in the latter the reverse is the case. Neurotic complaints arise from subconscious motives and can be treated by making the subject aware of these. In the case of the patient suffering from psychosomatic fatigue and pseudoneurosis, or false neurosis, there is no such motivation and he is best treated by rest and reassurance. He does not need analytical treatment and his complexes should not be laid bare.

> Every individual keeps hidden in his subconscious childish conflicts, which he has more or less mastered, which do not trouble him and which are not responsible for his exhausted condition. It would be a serious mistake to call up these shades and make a neurotic out of a nervous, exhausted individual. To avoid this danger it is necessary to appreciate the difference between exhaustion and neurosis, which can both present such similar clinical pictures. It is senseless to try and attribute the condition of an exhausted worker to his oedipus complex. Human relationships can be the cause of neurotic conflicts, but they cannot all be reduced to sexual terms, and unconscious conflicts are not among the main causes of fatigue in the world today.

8

*

Fatigue: A New Interpretation

SAMUEL BUTLER is reported to have written 'Life is one long process of getting tired.' The symptom of fatigue is ubiquitous and, although we cannot explain it to our satisfaction, neither can we forget about it or push it away into a dark cupboard. It will keep reminding us painfully that it exists and affect us, whether we choose to admit it or not. Despite the denials of scientists, many of us consider that it seriously influences our health and our ability to be productive. Without it, we feel well and cheerful. With it, we feel ill, morbid in our thoughts and powerless in our actions.

We will try in the following pages to show that fatigue is indeed real, capable of objective measurement and a precursor of some common debilitating illnesses and that it need not be accepted as inevitable.

In 1947 one of us (A.P.) saw two cases which made a deep impression and started an interest in the link between fatigue and disease. The first was a woman who came into hospital with a severe, painful and disabling rheumatoid arthritis. She was a pleasant, intelligent and conscientious person and she told her story without self-pity or exaggeration. For a year she had nursed an invalid father dying of some chronic disease – nursed him tenderly, lovingly, unremittingly; prepared to help at all times of the day or night, never asking neighbours or nurses to come to her aid. She felt exhausted, but had expected this and it did not deflect her from her duty. At some point towards the end of her father's illness, however, her arthritis had started insidiously and then gathered momentum.

The other patient was a man in his early thirties, who was learning to be a taxi driver and who, in the course of his training had to explore London by bicycle, getting to know and memorize every street. One day he had an almighty row with his wife and in his fury, and perhaps in his desire to escape from this situation, he had taken his bicycle and ridden the streets all night. Here it must be added that he had paid no attention to a sore throat he had contracted ten days to a fortnight earlier, which turned out to be relevant to what happened next. He returned home exhausted and a few days later was admitted to hospital with rheumatic fever. The sore throat had been a streptococcal infection, a necessary precursor of this dreadful disease, which in those days almost inevitably damaged the valves of the heart and usually resulted in invalidism. These two histories, both tragic and dramatic, appeared to be more than coincidental. It seems that exhaustion had in some way played a major part in the development of these rheumatic complaints.

Before discussing the experiments which were carried out to understand the nature of fatigue and to determine its influence on disease let us briefly review one or two aspects of fatigue and define some of the terms we shall be using. We should distinguish at once between acute, short term, natural fatigue and chronic fatigue. The former occurs at the end of the day or after strenuous physical or mental exertion. It is usually neither unpleasant nor unexpected and it is actually a help in inducing sleep which revives body and mind and chases fatigue away. In acute fatigue, we recognize a mental component, which must surely be due to brain cell fatigue and which can be resolved only by sleep; and a muscle component, related to depletion of resources and accumulation of breakdown products in the tissue which are restored by simple rest. This sort of fatigue is usually harmless if not carried to extremes and ill health rarely appears to follow.

The latter – chronic fatigue – is a different proposition. The subjective feeling of chronic fatigue is not one of simple brain and muscle tiredness after strenuous exertion. Indeed it is present day after day unprovoked by hard work. The whole body is pervaded by a lethargy, a disinclination to activity. The brain is muddled, numbed without having made an effort. There is bodily discomfort and a feeling of ill health. The point we wish to make is that acute fatigue is physiological and in most cases harmless, while chronic fatigue may have a pathological element about it which could lead to disease and deserves study to confirm whether this is true.

Conventional criticism at this stage will hold that chronic fatigue is the *outcome* of illness and not the precursor. There is some truth in this objection, but only partial truth. The assumption is made that a patient suffering from heart failure, bronchitis or a febrile illness is fatigued and this may of course be so, because of pain or sleeplessness or exertion beyond his capacity, but it is not invariably so. As we picture a man with heart failure we see him slowly moving his swollen legs, panting at the least exertion. Yet if he has slept well and is not in pain we will find him mentally alert and able to carry out light tasks efficiently. We are probably confusing shortness of breath and muscular weakness with fatigue, and this applies to many other illnesses. On the other hand there are some diseases in whose development fatigue probably does play a part, and in these conditions fatigue remains a symptom and may even increase in severity as the illness progresses.

The important point in the relationship between fatigue and disease is this. Does fatigue precede the disease in question or does it accompany or follow it? If it can be shown that it precedes a group of diseases then there is a possibility that it could be partly responsible for their development.

There were several pointers to the nature of chronic fatigue. The most striking of these was Addison's disease which has already been described in an earlier chapter (2, p 10). As has been said these patients suffer from a destruction of the adrenal gland. There is a deficiency of cortisol and the skin becomes pathologically pigmented. These poor people are desperately tired. If any one suffers from chronic fatigue, it is they. If, then, there should be a similarity between an Addisonian patient and other people suffering from chronic fatigue, we might expect that the latter will, in a minor way, exhibit some of the findings of Addison's. We should certainly look for relative cortisol insufficiency and a tendency to excess pigmentation.

Other pointers are given to us by circumstances attendant upon the discovery and use of cortisol and ACTH. Both drugs are, on occasion, used in the treatment of the severe Rheumatic ailments. As time passed, we found however, that this treatment is far from an unmitigated blessing and so we do our best to reduce dosage and discontinue treatment altogether when possible. What happens? There may be several withdrawal symptoms including – joint pains, nausea, headache and fatigue.[1] When, on the other hand, patients who suffer from Rheumatoid Arthritis and fatigue are given steroids, fatigue tends to subside.[2] Here again we seem to see a link between insufficient blood cortisol and fatigue.

The work of Selye has been of great value in relating non-specific stress to fatigue. You might like to refer back to the chapter on Selye and review his General Adaptation Syndrome (GAS) with its three stages, the second being the stage of resistance and the third, the stage of exhaustion. Come to think of it, there could be several reactions to stressful experience. The subject may not be able to adapt at all and succumbs immediately (the so-called stage of shock). He may adapt and cope indefinitely, or only for a limited time, in which case he may eventually fail as a result of exhaustion. This is the sort of commonsense approach Selye was trying to teach. How is it that we could not appreciate that human beings could fail because of a depletion of resources? Are we that invincible? Why be ashamed of failure through fatigue? Somehow we seem able to acknowledge only reversible acute fatigue and cannot bring ourselves to take chronic fatigue and chronic failure seriously, and we cannot imagine that this state could lead to disease.

Selye considered that a derailment of the second stage, that of resistance, was responsible for some diseases of adaptation; that an excess of mineralo-corticoid would result in high blood pressure, rheumatoid arthritis and polyarteritis (an allergic disease of arteries). He did not envisage a link between the rheumatic disorders and the stage of exhaustion. Our view, on the other hand, is that a modified, milder state of exhaustion is the real culprit in the rheumatic diseases, that excess of mineralo-corticoid is not implicated, but that relative cortisol insufficiency probably is.

We must also be grateful for the imaginative work which has been done on the Cluster Theory of Disease. Clusters of stressful life changes may result in clusters of diseases. This is now a fact which cannot be denied. Yet between the stressful events and the disease there must stretch an observable chain of physical events. Either the resistance of the body to disease is somehow lowered or an excessive reaction to strain results in some physiological adaptive process becoming pathological. It is reasonable to suppose that chronic fatigue is one of the channels through which maladaptation takes place – a failure of our energy resources.

For the moment, fatigue is a symptom, and until we have tied it down to some organs or functions in the body, it shall remain just a symptom. Meanwhile let us see what had happened to other symptoms. The ancients were at a loss to explain the cause of central chest pain, radiating to the arms. We know now that it is due to an insufficiency of oxygen reaching the heart muscle because of a narrowing of the coronary blood vessels. The symptoms of myxoedema (a condition in which the thyroid gland is underactive) – sluggishness of mind and body and an increased sensitivity to cold – were not understood until it was demonstrated that a deficiency of thyroid hormone was the cause. A host of other symptoms such as gall bladder colic, renal colic and sciatica were unexplained and incomprehensible until the underlying pathological processes were worked out. So it is with chronic fatigue. Today it is a mystery. Tomorrow it may have a meaning. We suggest it will come to be associated with relative cortisol insufficiency, just as the symptoms of myxoedema have come to be associated with thyroid deficiency.

How does a person develop chronic fatigue? The obvious causes are lack of sleep, persistent overwork and chronic anxiety. The anxious person does not rest mentally; he lives in a world of continual threat and danger and undoubtedly consumes an excess of mental energy. The less obvious causes of fatigue are the virus infections such as flu, glandular fever and infectious hepatitis, which in many cases are followed by a period of chronic fatigue and depression. There is indeed evidence that cortisol output is diminished in the post influenzal state. There may be other causes, for example nutritional.

Let us now set out our hypothesis linking chronic fatigue with disease and then see what evidence we have to support it. A person develops chronic fatigue as a result of factors mentioned above. The pituitary-adrenal axis becomes less responsive either because of decreased cerebral or hypothalamic activity, or sluggishness of the adrenal cortex itself. This results in a relative insufficiency of cortisol, ie relative to the subject's needs. Once the protective action of cortisol is removed certain consequences may follow and these will depend on the subject's hereditary and constitutional make up and harmful elements in the environment such as viruses, bacteria and chemicals. He may, for example, have a familial tendency to allergy or a predisposition to connective tissue disease. It should be remembered that cortisol has an anti-inflammatory and anti-allergic effect. If these actions of cortisol are not fully carried out, the door may be thrown open to inflammation of a rheumatic kind and to allergic reactions. We also know that cortisol will inhibit the thymus and lymphatic tissue and damp down antibody production by these elements. In the absence of sufficient cortisol, therefore, and under appropriate circumstances, antibodies could be produced, which would be harmful to the subject's own tissues. In these ways it is pictured that chronic fatigue may permit rheumatic disorders and allergies to develop.

It may seem rather naïve to put forward such a hypothesis. These ideas have, of course, been considered by others, considered and rejected for apparent lack of evidence. No one has consistently found low levels of cortisol in connective tissue diseases or allergies. We should not be put off by this, for several reasons. Firstly, we tend to label everyone without obvious disease as normal. This, to our mind, is untrue. The majority of the population is, of course, normal and healthy but some do live below par and suffer from chronic fatigue, without having yet developed any disease. At present such debilitated people are included in our concept of what is normal. If, as we suspect, they turn out to have lower cortisol levels then, by their exclusion, our range of normal cortisol values rises and we will cease to regard them as entirely normal but rather as a group which is 'at risk'. Secondly, we should study the early stages of disease when the severity of the disease has not yet distorted the circadian (twenty-four hour) rhythm of cortisol levels. When a disease is established, more cortisol is produced by the body, in an effort to damp down the illness. Hence we should expect to find normal or even high levels of plasma cortisol in severe asthma or active rheumatoid arthritis. But these levels are still not sufficient to do the job, for an intravenous injection of cortisol will calm the disease process temporarily and make the patient more comfortable. Lastly, we must take account of the whole circadian output. Adequate morning levels may not indicate a sufficiency towards the end of the day. This is precisely the relevant point. In our view, the fatigued person will not have a sufficient level of cortisol in the evening to give him the full protection he needs.

By now you will be getting tired of speculation and will be

asking for some evidence. There follow four experiments (carried out by A.P.) which provide some tangible results in support of these ideas. A study was carried out in 1959 on a 'healthy' population of doctors and nurses to show that this was not a uniform, homogeneous group but that it consisted, on the one hand, of really fit people not tiring excessively and, on the other, less fit subjects tiring well before the end of the day and that there were objective measurements which could be related to fatigue and which corresponded to the degree of fatigue. At that time estimations of cortisol in the blood were difficult and costly to carry out and so indirect methods were used to demonstrate activity of the adrenal cortex. Fortunately there were two simple means at hand. It was known that cortisol decreases the number of eosinophil cells in the blood. The eosinophil is a type of white blood cell which seems to have a special role in allergy. It stands out with certain stains and can be easily identified and counted.

Another indirect means of estimating adrenal cortex function is by measurement of capillary resistance (CR). The walls of tiny capillary blood vessels will, under normal circumstances, prevent leakage of red blood cells and this capacity or strength of the vessel walls is called the resistance. If the CR is high, then blood is retained, if it is low, cells are allowed to escape. Various factors can influence the CR. For instance, a dietary deficiency of vitamin C, as was so often the case in sailors on long distance voyages before the days of Captain Cook, will result in weakness of the capillaries and haemorrhages into the skin, while addition of vitamin C will strengthen them. Cortisol has a similar effect on capillaries and the CR rises with an increase in cortisol and falls with its decrease. As one might expect, the circadian CR curve follows the pattern of cortisol's curve.

There are two ways of bursting the capillary wall and causing minute haemorrhages into the skin. One is by binding a tourniquet around the upper arm, obstructing the return flow of blood through the veins and raising the pressure in the capillaries. The other, and more accurate way (employed in this experiment), is to apply a small suction cup to a greased area of the skin, thus lowering the pressure outside the capillary wall and achieving the same result.

These two methods were used to make an indirect assessment of adrenal cortex activity in the 'guinea pigs'. In this particular experiment, an attempt was made to link acute, short term fatigue with objective measurements and the task was to define the condition in an acceptable manner and divide it into its various grades of severity. Human fatigue is an amalgam of mental and physical components. Yet the boundary between these two factors is indistinct making it difficult, if not impossible, to evaluate their relative importance and so no attempt was made to separate the one from the other. Although fatigue is a subjective feeling a measure of objectivity can be introduced by reference to a framework of activity and efficiency. In this way we can describe four grades of acute fatigue (AF).

Grade one, no AF.	Not tired.
Grade two, mild AF.	a little tired, but work efficiency unimpaired.
Grade three, moderate AF.	more tired, work efficiency impaired.
Grade four, severe AF.	tired to such a degree that the subject feels the need to rest.

Fifty healthy colleagues agreed to enter the trial after it had been explained that the procedures were almost pain free and that there would be a sherry party when the whole experiment was over. Each subject was asked to place himself or herself in the right grade of AF, both morning and evening, after the definitions had been carefully explained. Tests were carried out at 9.30 am and 5.30 pm during the course of a normal working day during which they were asked not to smoke, drink alcohol or take pain killers which might all have distorted the results.

The experiment worked out well. Luckily about half of the subjects, in fact twenty-eight of them, experienced no increase of fatigue and were used as controls. It will be remembered that the circadian curve of CR normally shows a morning rise and an evening fall while that of the eosinophil cell count does the reverse and these were indeed the findings for the group as a whole.

But, and this is the significant point, there was a difference between those who were tired at the end of the day and those who were not. We found that the fall in the CR was nearly three times greater and the rise in the eosinophils was even more marked in the fatigued subjects.[3]

In healthy people, these findings are in keeping with the hypothesis that fatigue is associated, in part, with relative adrenocortical insufficiency. If this work is correct and can be reproduced, then we have at last the beginning of an approach to the objective measurement of fatigue. Once it can be measured it can no longer be regarded as a figment of the imagination, an excuse for laziness, a purely psychological phenomenon indicating boredom. What is more, we should be able to prove beyond doubt that fatigue is a precursor of some important diseases.

In this experiment the issue has been oversimplified and attention has been directed to only one aspect of fatigue – which seemed to be the most important – the functioning of the pituitary-adrenal axis, and some evidence has been produced to show that acute fatigue at the end of the day, is linked with decreased activity of this axis. But it is fully realized that the state of fatigue is not to be explained in quite so simple a way and that it will be found to be much more complex and to involve a myriad of subtle biochemical changes in the central nervous system, the endocrine glands and many other tissues and organs in the body. Nevertheless one can now speculate, with a little more assurance, on one chain of events in acute fatigue. Surely there is an element of brain cell fatigue, particularly of cells in the region of the hypothalamus. This in turn will lead to inadequate stimulation of the anterior pituitary, a decreased production of ACTH and diminished activity of the adrenal cortex. Yet none of these areas will show any structural change. It is only a question of impaired function which should be reversible.

9

*

Fatigue: Profile and Further Research

IN THE LAST CHAPTER, an attempt was made to show that acute fatigue is not a purely subjective phenomenon, but is associated with bodily changes which are measurable and which are in keeping with relative adrenocortical insufficiency. It has not been claimed, nor is it thought likely, that acute fatigue is a common precursor of illness. Analysis of case histories and common sense however, point to chronic fatigue having a more sinister meaning. Long continued fatigue, relentlessly lowering the ability of the subject to defend himself against a host of traumatic influences, is surely implicated in the development of some chronic diseases; if it could be shown that it is really a major factor in these conditions, we should have an important weapon in the battle against them. Impressions and feelings are not enough. Painstaking objective studies have to be carried out.

A study on hospital outpatients was carried out in the years 1957 to 1962, to see what objective differences could be found between patients suffering from chronic fatigue and controls and to discover whether this state was associated with a particular group of diseases. In all eighty-seven patients suffering from chronic fatigue and sixty-two controls, aged between twenty-five and sixty-five, were examined. The two groups were unfortunately not strictly comparable for age and sex as it is difficult to find tired young men and energetic old ladies but the average age of the controls was only a little less (three and a half years) than that of the chronic fatigue group and so some comparisons can be made.

Chronic fatigue may be defined as that fatigue which is not put right by the patient's normal hours of sleep and which continues for days or weeks on end. Like acute fatigue it can be subdivided into four stages, the basis of the subdivision depending upon work efficiency and inclination for social activity.

CFO: Not suffering from CF and able to work and take part in social activity without undue effort.
CF1: Able to carry out these activities, but with some effort and noticeable fatigue.
CF2: Able to work but with some impairment of efficiency. Disinclined to take part in social activity because of fatigue.
CF3: Work efficiency significantly impaired. Little or no social activity.

As was expected patients in the chronic fatigue group tended to suffer from a minor degree of insomnia. Both the fatigued group and the controls spent about eight hours in bed but the former lost half an hour's actual sleep and many tried to compensate for this by an equivalent period of daytime rest.

Bearing in mind that pigmentation of the skin occurs in Addison's disease where the adrenal gland is severely damaged it was not surprising that it was three times more common in the fatigued subjects and could be observed in as many as ten per cent of these patients.

It had been forecast that the rheumatic disorders would be more common in the fatigued group. There was some support for the prediction. The big toe joint served as an index of arthritis and was found to be deformed (hallux valgus) or stiff (hallux rigidus) in no less than seventy per cent of the fatigued subjects. In controls it was similarly affected in only thirty per cent. Another pointer was the frequency of a bowed or twisted spine. This was eight times more common in the fatigued group. In the rheumatic disorders painful 'fibrositic' nodules may sometimes be felt in the muscles of the shoulder girdle or deep under the skin of the lower back. These painful nodules were found in six per cent of the fatigued subjects but not at all in the controls.

Tiny capillary blood vessels tend to be more fragile when blood levels of cortisol are low and as pressure builds up in them they will leak red blood cells. Capillary fragility was measured by a rough method using a tourniquet and was found to be greater in the fatigued patients. One counts the number of blood spots (petechiae) per square centimetre. In the fatigued group this came to seven while in the controls it was only four. Muscle fatigue was assessed by squeezing an inflated cuff linked to a mercury gauge. Needless to say it was greater in the fatigued group.

Laboratory findings were again consistent with the hypothesis

TABLE II

Diseases Predominantly Affecting Fatigued Subjects

	Disease	*Control*	*Fatigue*
A)	Of General Nature		
	Peptic Ulcer (Duodenal and Gastric)	22	9
	Valvular Disease of Heart	3	3
	High Blood Pressure	2	4
	Coronary Insufficiency	2	4
B)	Of Connective Tissue		
	Rheumatoid Arthritis	0	8
	Osteoarthritis	0	3
	Prolapsed Intervertebral Disk	0	12
	Bursitis	0	2
	Gout	0	1
	Fibrositis	0	5
	Capsulitis Shoulder	0	1
	Reiter's Disease	0	1
C)	Of Undetermined Etiology		
	Raynaud's Phenomenon	0	3
	Median Nerve Compression	0	3
	Ménière's or Postural Vertigo	0	4

of relative insufficiency of the adrenal cortex. There were thirty-five per cent more eosinophil cells in the bloodstream of the fatigued patients and the chloride content was smaller. It will be remembered that Selye had noted a lowering of serum chlorides in his stage of exhaustion of the GAS.

One of the main purposes of this study was to discover which diseases commonly follow on the state of chronic fatigue. A glance at Table II gives the answer to this question. Most frequently encountered diseases in medical out-patients clinics, for example peptic ulcer, high blood pressure and angina of effort, were fairly evenly distributed between the fatigued patients and controls, and one can therefore assume that chronic fatigue played no significant part in their development. But connective tissue diseases stood out in that they were to be found only in the chronic fatigue group and not in the controls. This finding should not be exaggerated and common sense dictates that although osteoarthritis and gout were absent from the controls in this series there is no reason why a mainly traumatic condition – osteoarthritis – and a mainly metabolic condition – gout – should not occur in a non-fatigued group.

Three other conditions were found in the chronic fatigue group and not in controls: Raynaud's phenomenon in which the fingers go dead and blue in the cold; Ménière's disease where there is vertigo and a high-pitched singing noise in the ear; and compression of a nerve in the wrist giving rise to tingling and numbness in some fingers especially in the early morning.

No mention has been made of allergic disorders such as asthma. These conditions were not dealt with in the particular clinic but from experience in other departments and in general practice one can be confident that chronic fatigue plays a part in precipitating or aggravating many allergic illnesses.

Assuming then that chronic fatigue is associated with the rheumatic and allergic disorders we must still demonstrate that it precedes these conditions and may therefore be among the factors responsible for them. In the forty-three patients suffering from the rheumatic disorders and allied conditions fatigue was found to precede the illness by an average of fifteen months. This accords with the Cluster Theory of Disease, in which it has been shown that a cluster of stressful experiences precedes a cluster of illnesses.

If chronic fatigue is not just a nuisance but a possible precursor of illness can anything be done for the fatigued subject apart from such simple measures as increased sleep? Alcohol and tobacco have long been used to give pleasure, to remove inhibitions and to act as stimulants. Few are aware that they both increase blood cortisol levels and may therefore combat fatigue by reason of this action. As both these drugs are addictive and dangerous their routine use as stimulants is not advisable and it would be interesting to see whether other, less harmful, drugs could be found to fill the gap. Some research into this problem was carried out in general practice. The antidepressant Nortriptyline was used to see if it would counteract fatigue and influence blood levels of cortisol. This drug increases communication between brain cells by making serotonin and noradrenaline more available in the clefts between them. Perhaps the more active brain cells would stimulate the pituitary-adrenal axis. The trial was arranged on a double-blind basis with neither doctor nor patient knowing whether dummy or active capsules were being used. Twenty patients suffering from chronic fatigue very kindly took part. Fifteen of these reported a lessening of their fatigue after one month's treatment. Objective tests confirmed a change in pituitary-adrenal activity. The difference between morning and evening blood cortisol narrowed (from 6 units or micrograms to 3.6 units) and similarly the gap between morning and evening eosinophil counts and capillary resistance closed considerably. Muscle strength improved. A rather unexpected finding was that blood cortisol dropped both morning and evening, perhaps pointing to a decrease in the level of anxiety and to decreased need for cortisol. There are some disadvantages attached to this type of drug such as dryness of the mouth, constipation and possible serious consequences of overdose. We may therefore not be justified in using the antidepressants to counteract fatigue, but one can be sure that effective, non-addictive and non-toxic stimulants will soon be developed which will help the weary to face their everyday tasks with greater energy and cheerfulness.

A final experiment, which brings us a little nearer to proof of an association between chronic fatigue and a low blood cortisol, must be reported. It was carried out in General Practice in the years 1976 to 1979. Twenty-five cases of chronic fatigue were matched for age and sex with twenty-five controls. 9 a.m. blood cortisol levels were determined with the help of the department of steroid biochemistry at Hammersmith Hospital. As predicted the average blood cortisol level in the fatigued subjects (Table III) was statistically lower than in controls.[1]

TABLE III

Plasma Cortisol in Chronic Fatigue

	Plasma Cortisol in micrograms per 100 millilitres	
	Control	*Fatigue*
9.00 a.m.	15.0	11.8

Twenty-five pairs of patients matched for age and sex

In the course of this work an attempt was made to search for a link between chronic fatigue and the psychosocial environment. Each patient was asked to complete a social readjustment rating questionnaire which has been described in the chapter on the Cluster Theory of Disease. On average the number of life change units scored by the chronic fatigue group was 117 while controls scored only sixty-nine units. This takes account of the results in the increased number of participants in the trial.

What then is the significance of these observations on acute and chronic fatigue? Illness does not develop of its own accord but because of maladaptation or malfunctioning of our protective mechanisms. We need a well-balanced mind, sound organs to perform the day-to-day tasks of the body and we need energy. This last factor has not been taken sufficiently into account in orthodox medical teaching and this is understandable as we have tended to think in terms of simple muscle energy, fuelled by sugar or fat, to perform physical work. There are, however, many other forms of energy which are complex and less well-defined. Do we need 'fuels' to enable brain cells to work, to activate our endocrine glands, to control our defence mechanisms and regulate inflammatory reactions? It has always been assumed that we are all capable of producing enough energy to meet these demands. But this is probably a false assumption and we should study derailment of the adaptive process (as Selye has done) and energy deficits. We do not yet know what these missing energy substances are.

They might be neurotransmitters. They might be high energy phosphates (such as cyclic AMP) which act as 'second messengers' and prod the cell into activity after it has been stimulated from outside by the 'first messenger' (usually a hormone such as adrenaline). Whatever the nature of the energy factor we can postulate from the work here described that energy depletion is associated with low levels of blood cortisol.

So we must learn to take the symptom of fatigue, or lack of energy, seriously and recognize that it is associated with cortisol insufficiency, that if allowed to continue it will lead, sooner or later, to disease in a high proportion of cases. One in twenty of the population will, at some time or other, have a serious allergic complaint and at least a further one in ten will suffer from a serious connective tissue disease. We are all aware of the suffering and invalidism brought about by asthma and rheumatoid arthritis. In our view these conditions are often preventable and when they occur they should respond to energetic and imaginative treatment in the early stages of the disease provided one recognizes the significance of chronic fatigue.

Let us consider prevention of the illnesses which arise from fatigue. A patient may complain that he is continually tired and ask what can be done for him, or he may produce a lot of minor symptoms and later agree, on questioning, that he is also very tired. The doctor has a way of disregarding, almost not hearing, symptoms for which he has no explanation and no cure. So apart from a blank look or a mildly sympathetic smile he may get no response. But, in the new era, where fatigue will not be brushed aside and will be taken seriously, the physician will take a detailed history and make a full examination to try to get to the bottom of this, now important, symptom. A review of the patient's mental state and his social and interpersonal background may throw light on the causes of his fatigue; or he may have had a virus infection from which he has not fully recovered. Only rarely will no cause be found. It is of course possible that the symptoms will be due to existing illness such as anaemia, chronic kidney disease, cancer and so on, and these conditions must obviously be looked for and treated. Here the fatigue is secondary.

The type of action which is needed when primary fatigue has been found depends on the seriousness of the overall condition. If no threat of significant connective tissue disease or allergy looms on the horizon simple discussion and advice may meet the bill. If there should be symptoms of early rheumatoid arthritis, for example, then active measures must be taken to deal with the situation giving rise to fatigue and to treat the arthritis. A case history illustrates the point. A young woman, whose mother is almost an invalid with severe rheumatoid arthritis which has necessitated the use of steroids and surgery, attends the consulting room with obvious early rheumatoid arthritis affecting hands, wrists and knees. She tires easily and requires a lot of sleep. She has already been treated with physiotherapy and large doses of aspirin. We know she might progress to the same degree of invalidism as her mother and she, too, is well aware of this. It is at this point, when damage is minimal, that we must move heaven and earth to arrest the disease. The physician will want to establish a warm sympathetic relationship and listen patiently to a detailed biographical story. He will hear of the parents' attitude to her from infancy and the way each relationship grew. He will form an idea of the child's character and personality and discover her weaknesses and vulnerable areas, her capabilities and ambitions, her successes and failures and the traumatic events in her life. Then comes a formulation. The physician, without pretending to understand and interpret all things, will try to explain to the patient the development both of her fatigue state and of her illness and the association between them. He will discuss with her the link between her personality and her reaction to experience and the development of fatigue through unresolved emotional problems. He will go on to describe some of the body's defences against illness and how the internal production of cortisol will damp down the activity of rheumatic inflammation and point out that fatigue is associated with a low blood cortisol which is harmful. The fatigue state can be improved by understanding and solving one's emotional problems. First 'know thyself' then 'heal thyself.'

There are two useful mental pictures which help the patient. The first (Fig. VIII) is to imagine the brain as a battery which is healthy when fully charged. It will then be able to stimulate the pituitary which, in turn, stimulates the adrenal. The battery may be run down by emotional distress and recharged by adequate sleep and solution of problems. The second (Fig. IX) is a diagram of a normal blood cortisol curve. Set against this, is one which

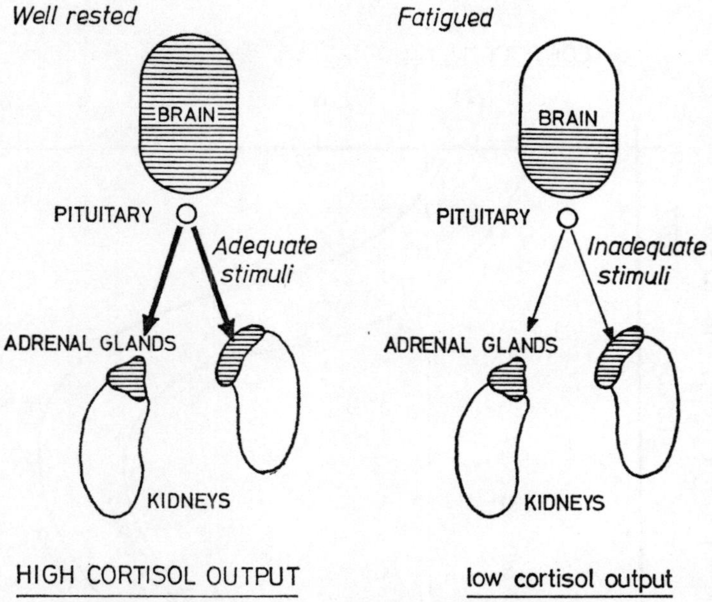

Fig VIII. Fatigue and adrenal activity, (postulated)

might occur in fatigue.

If the patient were a paragon of wisdom and behaviour she would probably not be in the situation she is in, so that simple explanation is not likely to fall on totally receptive ears. She may, with her intelligence, see the logic of the argument and the need to follow the offered advice but, with all the good will in the world, she will not be able to carry out the ideal programme. How can a young person go to sleep early, how can she isolate herself from traumatic experiences, how can she readjust her inter-personal relationships to suit her need for peace and calm? But this should not put us off. The seed is sown, an explanation is offered. We must be hopeful that, over a period of time, the patient will be more capable of avoiding traumatic situations, of coping with existing problems and, in any event, making up for the emotional loss of energy by extra sleep.

At present we are not adjusted psychologically, administratively or financially to the prevention of the chronic rheumatic diseases. We wait until the disease is well established before we arrange

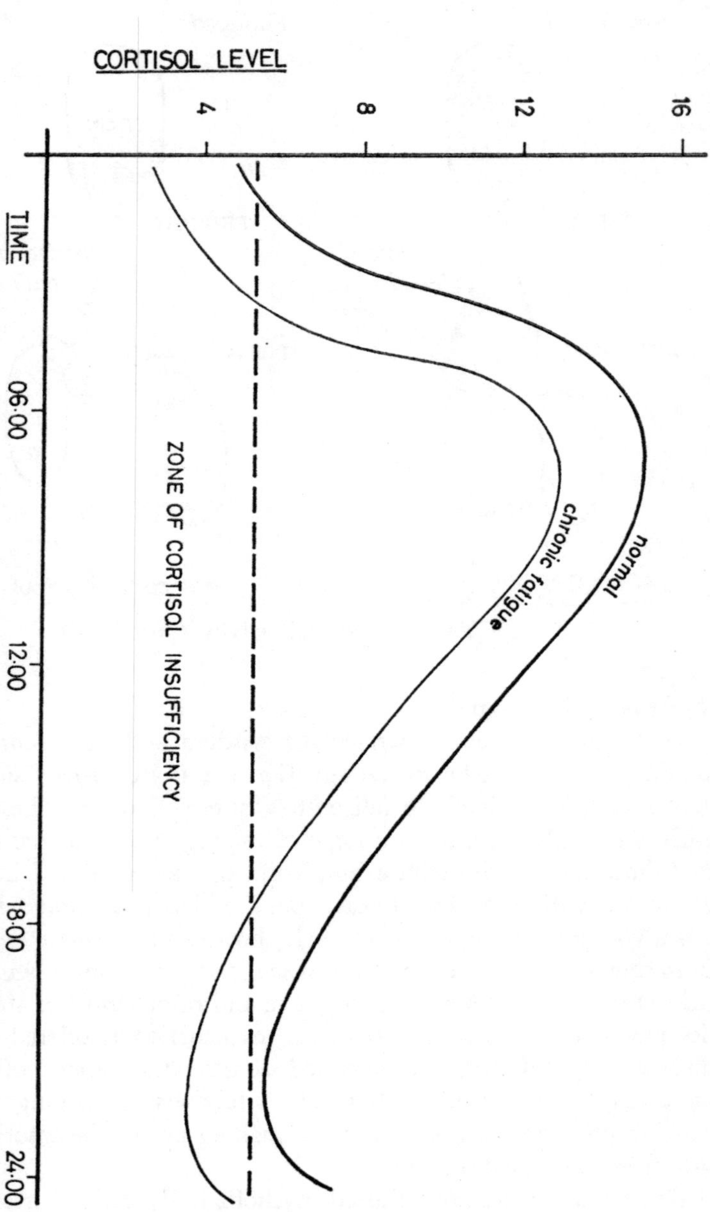

Fig IX. Blood cortisol (postulated) levels in normal and fatigued subjects

hospital admission for bed rest. We will discharge a patient who has made some progress back into the community where all the social and financial pressures fall on her before she is fully cured. It is therefore almost inevitable that a complete return to health is impossible, that there will be residual damage and deformity and that there will be a relapse of the disease process. So, in spite of good intentions, we have too many rheumatoid invalids who are a burden to themselves and to society.

The achievements of an intelligent and purposeful community can be seen in the field of tuberculosis prevention. It must be admitted that in addition to the high mortality at one time associated with the disease there was the danger of spread by contagion – so society was well motivated to its eradication. No effort was spared. On the mountain slopes of Switzerland, in the rolling countryside of all European countries sanatoria were built for both rich and poor. Chest clinics, giving free treatment, were established. Patients were kept in sanatoria for months or years where they either recovered or died. Not so with rheumatoid arthritis. Beds and resources are scarce. A sanatorium regime is rarely used. Yet we feel sure that most patients with this disease would recover if given all the resources society could muster, as was the case with the dread enemy, tuberculosis.

One of the main obstacles to adequate treatment is the attitude of patients themselves. They do not want to be deprived of their freedom to live a normal life and to be self-supporting. The attitude of the patient must therefore be changed concurrently with that of society and while the latter must be prepared to supply the resources, the former must be persuaded to accept them. If then, in spite of simple ambulant treatment, the patient's disease progresses he should be admitted to hospital or sanatorium where the right combination of treatment can be given and the patient be sheltered from the traumas, both interpersonal and financial, to which he is exposed in the community. It might take two months or it might take well over a year but, if it succeeds, then every effort made and every penny spent will have been worth it. This approach has not yet been applied except in special circumstances so we are not certain what would happen if we applied it. But if the theoretical reasoning is correct then we may be sure it will make a very substantial contribution to the management of these diseases. Certainly there are pointers to the correctness of this claim. The physician, George Ernest Beaumont, described the case of a very busy medical consultant who developed joint troubles during the last war when he worked around the clock. His colleagues advised physiotherapy but, as the condition rapidly deteriorated, he took matters into his own hands and rested for a period of some months, making a full recovery. Another case is of a girl medical student who contracted rheumatoid arthritis while studying for her exams. The arthritis progressed in spite of treatment and some wise physician ordered a sanatorium regime which, over a period of many months, halted the condition, but not before permanent deformities had set in.

We would not like to give the impression that rest is the only treatment. Far from it. There is a vast arsenal of agents – pain-killing and antirheumatic drugs, the occasional use of steroids in selected cases, preventive and corrective surgery in the occasional patient who resists medical treatment, physiotherapy and psychotherapy where needed. Total rest is both unnecessary and indeed dangerous. Muscles must be exercised and joints moved to retain function. The rest we are talking about is partly physical, but to a large extent it is mental. The patient should be sheltered by removing his anxieties. Where a housewife is admitted her family must be cared for and this is no cheap and easy task. Where a breadwinner is ill the family income cannot be allowed to drop appreciably and his commitments, be they of hire purchase or mortgage repayments, should be covered. Without this sort of provision no one will accept hospitalization for months on end and they will sacrifice long term health for present commitments. There is, to our mind, no better investment than in the health of individual members of a community. Think how much suffering and invalidism can be prevented in the long run, how much money can be saved on various benefits, such as home helps, district nurses, major surgery and invalid cars. The initial cost is enormous but long term savings will be high and you have a healthy, happy person into the bargain who remains productive in the community.

We do not expect the Medical Profession to accept the value of a sanatorium regime in rheumatoid arthritis and the general hypothesis of chronic fatigue in relation to the connective tissue diseases without further proof. Neither the profession nor the Government can be asked to invest great effort and large capital resources in projects which are not fully established. But serious research should be carried out to allow full assessment and firm decisions. We have the conviction that not only will rheumatoid arthritis respond to this approach but that, by health education, and making use of the model of chronic fatigue and disease, many of the rheumatic conditions can be prevented from occurring.

10

Sleep and Dreams

THE ACADEMIC CONSIDERATION of stress and fatigue, although interesting, is of little value unless the restorative and adaptive processes, which counteract these states, are likewise studied, understood and applied. Sleep is the pre-eminent healer and yet it has, for unaccountable reasons, been fashionable to minimize its importance. Both the medical profession and the lay public tend to hold rather extreme views on sleep. Some doctors will give a hypnotic drug too readily, either out of sympathy or else as a quick and superficial means of dealing with the patient's insomnia without the need to delve more deeply into its origins. If the choice of drug is not carefully undertaken addiction may result. Then there is the doctor who shrugs off the whole business. He may genuinely believe that loss of sleep is harmless and addiction is a greater evil. He will point to the fortunate few who lead perfectly normal lives in spite of limited sleep and he will insist that moderate sleep loss has not been known to impair mental efficiency or physical health. He may not wish to add anxiety to insomnia and make a hypochondriac of his patient. The unfortunate insomniac gets little comfort from these reassurances. He knows he is irritable, forgetful and has lost his usual sparkle of mind and clarity of thought. He feels off-colour and notices a gradual accumulation of minor illness.

Similarly the lay person is either a ready pill taker and insists on help the moment he experiences a poor night's sleep or he will stoically accept insomnia and nothing will make him swallow a pill which he regards as a poison.

In these attitudes little account is taken of the wide variation of human adaptability and human frailty. There are indeed a fortunate few who can manage perfectly well on four to six hours sleep a night, but there are others who are shattered by loss of even a small portion of their sleep. Some will remain physically healthy, others will break down into illness.

We need then a rational, balanced and flexible approach to insomnia based on understanding and adapted to the needs of particular individuals. Let us not sweep uncomfortable facts under the carpet but look at the situation objectively and scientifically.

The Cluster Theory of Holmes and Rahe has shown conclusively that a cluster of stressful events is followed by a cluster of illnesses and we have also seen that chronic fatigue has its own retinue of ill effects in the form of allergic and connective tissue disorders. It is becoming more obvious as time passes that loss of sleep and the ensuing chronic fatigue must be taken seriously and rectified. The task is not an easy one and requires an understanding of the nature of sleep and insomnia, of the means of inducing natural, wholesome sleep, avoiding, where possible, the use of drugs and unnecessary introspection and anxiety.

A good deal of material dealt with in this chapter comes from two excellent books. The first, *Concepts of Sleep*,[1] brought out by Roche in 1965, is a review of many aspects of sleep including its relationship to the arts. The second, published in 1969 and edited by Anthony Kales[2] is a report on a symposium on the subject, held by experts in the field, for the benefit of general physicians.

Sleep is a well organized process occurring mainly in the brain but involving most of the body systems. It is by no means a total shutdown of activity. The shop may be closed but all sorts of activities are going on inside. Stocktaking, repairing, cleaning, recharging of batteries, introduction of new stock ready for the day's needs and a host of other processes take place behind the shutters. The brain cells are not totally paralysed, nor do they all rest at the same time. At one moment the cortex of the brain, which can be regarded as the newer, intellectual component, is partially resting, while some time later, it is more active and the mid-brain, or primitive and emotional part of the brain rests in its turn. During sleep the parasympathetic predominates while during activity the sympathetic tends to do so.

Our knowledge of what goes on in sleep is derived from the many excellent studies that have been made in the last two or three decades in sleep laboratories using the Electro Encephalogram (EEG). A series of tiny metal electrodes are placed on the scalp, and weak electric currents on the surface of the brain are

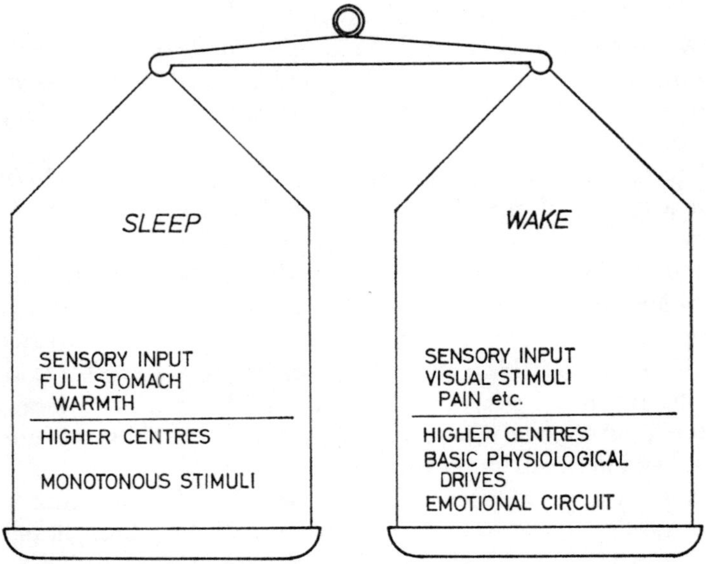

Fig X. Balance of forces in sleep and wakefulness

picked up, magnified and recorded on moving paper. It is at once obvious that sleep does not mean a cessation of brain activity but only an alteration of the type of activity.

A meshwork of brain tissue in the mid-brain, called the reticular system, is responsible for rousing the cerebral cortex into conscious activity. If this system is destroyed in the experimental animal, perpetual sleep results. If, on the other hand, it is stimulated, then perpetual wakefulness is generated.

There is an inherent circadian rhythm in the reticular system which can be modified both by stimuli from the cortex and by incoming stimuli from the main sensory tracts. At first sight there would appear to be many advantages if we could induce sleep in ourselves at will, as if we were turning off some electrical switch, and wake again by some simple device, but this is not how evolutionary forces have shaped us, for they have had to take into account the overriding requirement of defence of the organism as a whole, and so sleep can only occur with the assurance of safety.

There seems to be a balance of forces (Fig. X) that wake us and cause sleep and a tilt of that balance will bring us into one or other state. Tilting us towards the side of sleep are natural, mental and physical fatigue, an inbuilt circadian rhythm which influences the brain and endocrine system, darkness, warmth, satisfied hunger and sexual activity, repetitive words and music, various conditioned reflexes, alcohol and a host of soporific drugs, and possibly naturally occurring hormones which act on specific parts of the brain. On the side of wakefulness are arrayed the opposing factors – physical and mental energy (the body refreshed), the clamour of many instinctual drives such as the demand for food and safety, the inbuilt circadian clock which rouses us to activity, the many colourful sensations which bombard us and, finally, the emotions which are generated in us to affect the reticular system and maintain the drive for wakefulness and purposeful living.

The opposing forces are pitched against each other. Daytime usually sees the victory of wakefulness and night that of sleep but this is not invariably so and there are many occasions on which we have to fight an encroaching sleepiness by day or an unwelcome, intruding wakefulness by night.

If we were to pick out the main factors encouraging sleep we would probably point to healthy fatigue after satisfying mental or physical work, and a mind untroubled by anxiety. In contrast, factors encouraging wakefulness would be – a surplus of unused energy, a lack of satisfaction with the day's activity, anxiety, fears and pain.

Let us assume we have fulfilled all the conditions needed for sleep and our subject is about to enter that agreeable and mysterious kingdom. The knowledge gained in sleep laboratories will tell us about the stages of sleep and the mental and bodily activities which are to be found in each stage. Before actually entering sleep there is a state of relaxed wakefulness or drowsiness in which conscious thought is slipping away. There will be eye movements and blinking of the eyelids; muscle tone, or tension, which, as shown by the electro myogram is high. The EEG (Fig. XI) shows an α rhythm – fairly regular waves of medium height at about ten cycles per second. This passes into stage one of light sleep from which the subject can easily be roused. The eyes now show slow rolling movements. The EEG changes to a low voltage, mixed frequency pattern. In stage two the muscles are relaxed, but some muscle tone remains. Sleep spindles at twelve to fourteen cycles per second, appear on the EEG and here and there, taller, slower

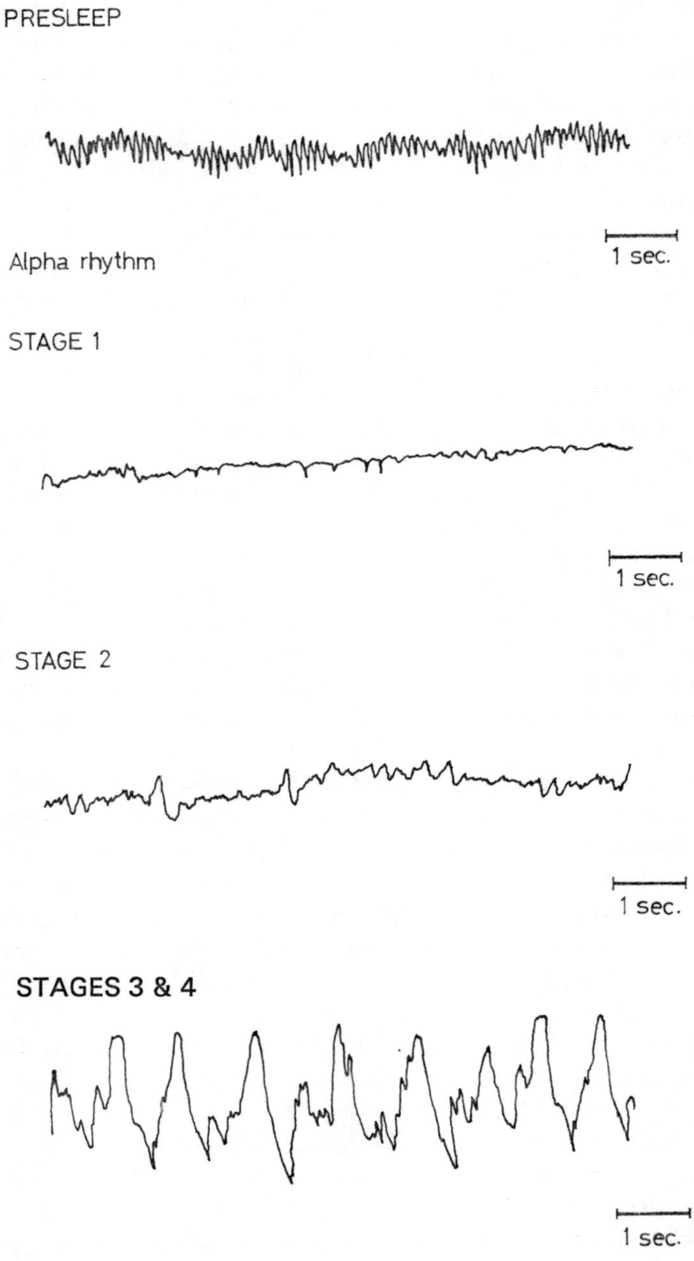

Fig XI. The Electroencephalogram in sleep

waves known as K complexes which may occur spontaneously or as a result of external stimuli, are to be seen. The subject passes into the deeper sleep of stage three and four in which slow, high voltage waves appear at one to two cycles per second.

An important and entirely distinct stage of sleep, not graced by any numeral, has so far not been mentioned. It is that of paradoxical or REM sleep, a lighter form of sleep in which the EEG resembles that of stage one but the Electro Myogram (EMG) (which depicts electrical activity in muscle) shows almost toneless muscles and the characteristic rapid eye movements are both visible and recordable (on the electro oculogram) and give to this form of sleep one of its strange titles.

The sleeper moves gradually through the various stages to reach stage four which is called orthodox or slow sleep on account of the tall slow waves which are recorded on the EEG tracing. He may remain on this level for about an hour and then move quickly upward to paradoxical or REM sleep in which he may stay for some twenty minutes before returning to orthodox sleep, and this pattern continues throughout the night. In this way the average sleeper passes through some four to six cycles of REM and non-REM sleep, each of approximately ninety minutes duration. Between fifteen and twenty-five per cent of all sleep will be spent as REM sleep.

The other description for REM sleep, ie 'Paradoxical', requires explanation. The meaning becomes clear when we consider the phenomena associated with it. Superficially this kind of sleep appears to be deep. The muscles are limp, the subject difficult to rouse. Yet this is deceptive, for the sleeper dreams and the EEG shows cortical activity which is akin to that found in wakefulness.

It would be tempting to think that rapid eye movements are the natural concomitant of dreaming and that the eyes are following an object seen in the dream, but this is not the case as the movements are not like those occurring in day-time vision, nor do they always happen concurrently with a dream. Their nature and purpose remain unsolved.

The reason for so complete a flaccidity and tonelessness of the muscles in REM sleep is the other enigma. Here, at least, we know something of the mechanism involved but not the purpose. In REM sleep the reticular system is out of action. It ceases to transmit impulses to the cortex. As it is also concerned with the

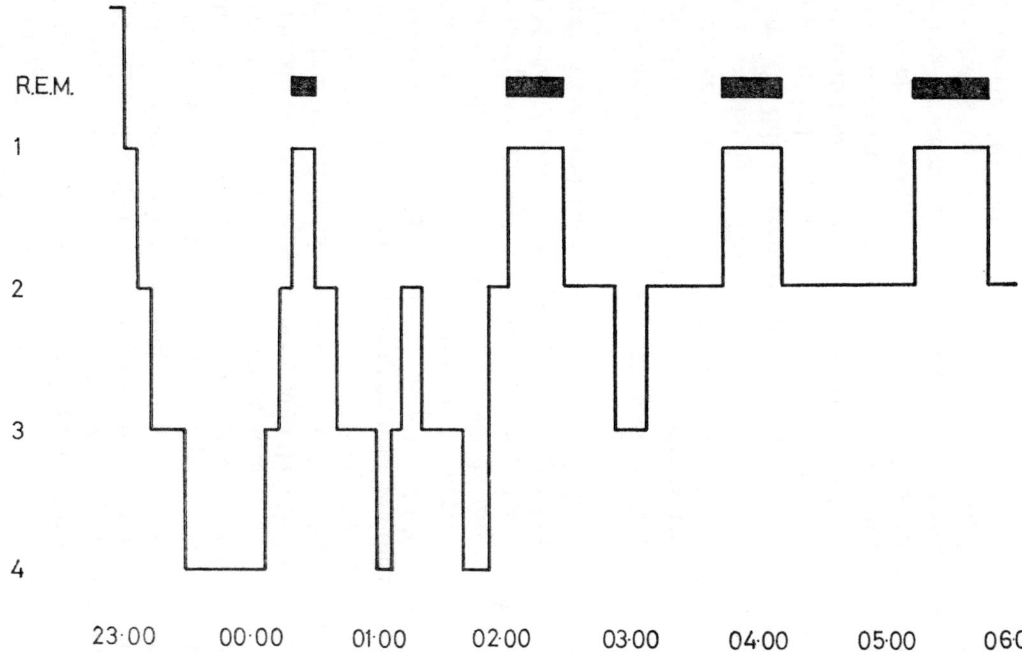

Fig XII. Sleep pattern showing alternating periods of non REM (orthodox) and REM (paradoxical) sleep. Thick bar represents periods of REMs

maintenance of muscle tone this is relinquished and the body becomes limp. It is in this stage of sleep that arousal of the subject is particularly difficult. One wonders whether nature has not insisted on loss of muscle tone in REM sleep. What would have happened otherwise? The subject engaged in one vivid dream after another would not just lie there passively but might easily get up and take an active role in the dream sequence, possibly chasing his bed fellow or himself fleeing from some monster. It seems just as well that we are paralysed at this stage. When we talk of paralysis we do not, of course, mean irreversible paralysis. A good shaking and the subject wakes. How many wives will shake their husbands, out of kindness, if they notice they are in some horrible nightmare, so as to let them escape from their terror. And then again, lack of movement in REM sleep cannot be absolute. It is essential in both this phase of sleep and in that of non REM sleep that gross body movements should occur from time to time or else long continued immobility would lead to pressure ulcers over bony points such as heels and buttocks, as may occur in comatose subjects. Provision has in fact been made for this and we find gross body movements taking place several times an hour in all phases of sleep.

The loss of tone in REM sleep is well illustrated by an experiment which has been carried out to prevent REM and gauge the ill-effects of deprivation. The animal is placed on a small raft in a pool of water. EEG wires are connected to the surface of the skull. As the typical EEG waves of REM sleep appear, the animal becomes limp and cannot help falling into the pool. As this experience is not very pleasant, it learns to avoid REM sleep, and so the results of the deprivation of this phase of sleep can be studied.

Recent laboratory work has led to a partial understanding of the biochemical mechanisms involved in sleep. There is evidence that 5 Hydroxytryptophan, a precursor of Serotonin, one of the biological amines found in the brain, encourages non REM sleep, while noradrenaline is needed to induce REM sleep. REM sleep does not, however, take place without a preceding non REM phase primed by Serotonin. It would indeed be dangerous for an animal to enter REM sleep, associated as it is with flaccidity and difficulty in arousal, without first undergoing a period of non REM sleep. These biochemical mechanisms involved in sleep production are, to say the least, very unexpected. Serotonin is usually thought of as being required for satisfactory brain function and many of the antidepressants act by increasing the available Serotonin; while noradrenaline is associated with the body's emergency response to threat or stress and so it is difficult to picture these two substances being concerned in the sleep process. Yet, on reflection, is not orthodox sleep a stage in the restoration of brain cell function and is not REM sleep the more active phase of sleep in which perhaps we are preparing to face emergency? We need not therefore be too surprised if Serotonin and noradrenaline, acting on circumscribed and specialized portions of the brain and liberated in minute quantities, play a role in the genesis of sleep.

We have touched on arousal during REM sleep but what about vigilance and arousal during all stages of sleep. In the animal world, exposed to constant danger, sleep must not be allowed to rob us of our defences. So arousal must be geared to the need for essential activity such as hearing a crying baby or rising in self-defence. Warning signals must be allowed to penetrate, as far as possible, to the centres which initiate activity. To a remarkable extent this is so. There is a selective vigilance, greatest in orthodox sleep but still available in paradoxical sleep. The mechanism is preset. The mother will hear only the noise of her infant's cry but ignore the cars in the street or footsteps on the stairs. The soldier will pick up a call to action but not the chatter and laughter of his comrades. Sleep is mercifully instantaneously reversed if the need arises and no one knows this better than the doctor whose mind can be totally alert in a second to deal with an emergency, or the fireman who can slide down a pole seconds after waking from any stage in sleep. So, like our hearts and lungs which never totally rest, our brains are never totally asleep but sentinels are posted and only portions of the brain are allowed to rest at any one time. Sometimes the cortex rests, sometimes the reticular system, but both are never rested together except in deep drug induced coma from which, of course, we cannot be roused.

Drugs can lower or raise the arousal threshold. Alcohol, sedatives and hypnotics render arousal more difficult, while drugs such as the amphetamines and caffeine make it easier. In a similar way different emotions influence arousal. Anxiety thwarts the onset of sleep and brings about easy arousal by prolonging the bombardment of the cortex. By contrast, calm and contentedness appear to depress the activity of the reticular formation.

A curious and useful phenomenon is the ability of some people to wake at a predetermined time. They will instruct themselves to wake at, say, 8.00 am and will do so. Others have the faculty but do not trust their natural clock and rely on the mechanical alarm clock.

Vigilance does not necessarily imply behavioural consciousness. Stimuli which are not meaningful may be totally ignored while those which are meaningful are assessed. If they are not threatening the EEG just records a transient response in the form of a particular kind of wave pattern, already referred to – the K complex. If the stimulus is judged to be theatening or requiring action the subject wakes. So our subconscious mind will do its work while the master sleeps – rousing him to action if predetermined situations arise.

REM sleep is associated with dreaming and this is easy enough to demonstrate as subjects woken in this phase of sleep, almost invariably admit to dream activity. This is the case to a far lesser extent in non REM sleep for only seven to ten per cent of subjects woken from this form of sleep will recall dreams. But why do we dream? Is it accidental or essential? The answer is not easy and is, at the moment, far from complete. We know, for example, that REM sleep is not essential for the reptile. He has none. It is infrequent in birds, occupying only some 0.2 per cent of total sleep. A bird sleeps perched on a branch and REM sleep, which involves loss of muscle tone, would be disastrous. So nature does not insist on it. A kitten at birth is engaged in REM sleep for ninety per cent of its sleeping time and gradually moves towards the normal ratio of REM to slow sleep. REM sleep in human beings appears to be essential. If deprived of it the loss will be made good when conditions allow. For example, if a subject is deprived of REM sleep for seventy-two hours then, on being allowed to sleep in an unrestricted way, he will indulge in REM sleep for sixty per cent of sleeping time as opposed to the usual twenty-five per cent. Deprivation of REM sleep is followed in most subjects by increased tension and anxiety, difficulty in concentration, disturbances of memory and increased irritability and hostility. In contrast deprivation of stage four of non REM sleep tends to lead to underactivity, lethargy and inadequate responses.

We may have established that REM sleep is essential but we must admit we do not fully know why this is so. There are numerous speculations. An acceptable proposition would be that the brain is brushing up the information it has, integrating it and reaching new sub-conscious concepts. It may be that without dreams the information we possess would fade even more quickly than it does. It is remarkable that most people can remember useful facts for some seven years. Trivial facts have a much shorter life, while facts which have at some time been associated with strong emotions are remembered in an imperfect way even for a lifetime. Dreams may help us to review impressions and to reimprint the more vivid and emotionally charged ones so as to prolong their lives.

That new ideas emerge out of dreams is common knowledge. Paul Ehrlich saw a reptile eating its own tail in a dream and woke with the solution of the chemical formula of the Benzene ring which happened to be a six-sided ring structure. Literature, poetry and painting are all indebted to the inspiration of dreams. Creativity consists in adding a new element or dimension to an existing concept or structure. How much easier it is to do this divorced from the painful need to conform to the hard reality of the day. One can picture the budding poet or writer, woken by the excitement of a wonderful vision, searching for pen and putting the fleeting thought upon paper.

The psychoanalyst may make use of the dream to understand his patient the better, but nature, unaware of him while tinkering with the development of the human mind over a million years, did not create the dream for his benefit. A glimpse of the analytical view of dreams may be had from the following extract from the *Concept of Sleep* –

> Freud's concept of the dream – as remembered by the sleeper (manifest content) – was of an elaborate and extravagant masquerade. It would be a collection of unconscious desires, wishes and impulses – all heavily disguised – of which the dream material (latent content) was really composed. In any undisguised form such unconscious material would be rejected by the conscious mind as quite unacceptable. But with appropriate disguises furnished by such dream mechanisms as symbolization, displacement, condensation and dramatization, the sleep of the dreamer would be assured. He would thus sleep on accepting, if puzzled by, the extraordinary stream of events which passed in his conscious mind . . .

Rather well put but is it true? The suggestion that the actual dream content is disguised to make it more acceptable is unconvincing. Our subconscious is not that considerate and submits a terrifying array of threatening, unpalatable material to us as dream food.

There may be an emotional gain from our dreams. Tensions may perhaps be resolved or lessened. Fear and anger may be acted out in dreams leaving us calmer in our waking state. There is, in fact evidence, as we have already seen, that deprivation of REM sleep is followed by increased irritability and aggressiveness.

Our understanding of one of the main functions of REM sleep is that it allows a state of semipreparedness at regular intervals throughout the night to enable us to cope with possible emergencies. In deep, orthodox sleep the cortex is almost totally idle and the mind a blank. It is conceivable that this would lead to a totally unprepared brain and body, if and when a threat came or dawn broke. But REM sleep warms up the engine. The car is still stationary and the engine has not been put into gear but it is ready to leap into action. This view is supported by the fact that Cortisol is produced during REM sleep and enters the bloodstream ready to support demands made on the body.

Sleep Loss

So much for REM sleep and dreams but we must not forget the totality of sleep – orthodox and paradoxical. What goes wrong when we don't get enough? Let us look at the extreme case first and then study the milder and more subtle deprivations. A total embargo on sleep is a known stresser of the human mind. This is well known to the torturer and the tortured. To the unutterable shame of both Western and Eastern countries, in fact almost wherever human beings exist, we will find aggression supported by the extortion of information by violent means. The more sophisticated torturers resort to less obvious and less tangible methods, such as sleep and sensory deprivation. The will to resist is broken, the mind confused and the confession extracted.

In animals prolonged sleep deprivation has led to actual physical damage to portions of the brain. Changes of degeneration have been found in the cortex and even in the reticular formation.

Human volunteers have been kept awake for ten or more days.

In the early stages they developed symptoms such as difficulty in focussing the eyes, nausea and memory losses. Later come irritability, fragmentation of sentences, slurred speech and, only occasionally, psychotic behaviour with, at times, hallucinations.

We need not concern ourselves too much with prolonged sleep deprivation as it is infrequently encountered. Less dramatic periods of sleep loss or substantial sleep debt are more common and these are naturally accompanied by fatigue. In addition there will be 'lapses' which might be microsleeps – short spells of inattention, thought is slowed down, reaction time is prolonged, memory is impaired. The subject is at his worst during the night and early morning, and better as the day wears on especially towards evening. This is in keeping with the body's natural circadian rhythm.

Efficiency is impaired, but not uniformly for all tasks. Work which is paced or directed by the experimenter is not as well performed as that which is self-directed. If a subject is asked to respond in a particular manner to a visual or auditory stimulus then errors of omission rather than of commission will occur and these will increase with the prolongation of sleep loss. If, on the other hand, the subject can perform tasks at his own pace, especially if he is well motivated, as for example, he would be if he is placed in command, then problem solving, issuing orders and making judgements will be moderately well carried out. Speed may be impaired but accuracy will be maintained.

Sleep loss or sleep debt are often not recognized by the subject because, strangely enough, a euphoria may impair self-assessment. In sleep deprived persons every effort is made to catch up a sleep debt and, given a chance, they will sleep well over their normal ration. The sleep of an exhausted person will contain a high proportion of the deeper stages three and four but the amount of REM sleep is also greater than normal.

The Physical Value of Sleep

Only in recent years has it come to be realized that sleep is needed not only for the restoration of the brain function, but also for the restoration of the body as a whole. In 1977 two eminent sleep researchers, Kirstine Adam and Ian Oswald published an article entitled 'Sleep is for Tissue Restoration'.[3] It explains the essential role of sleep in growth and restoration. It has been shown that sleep deprivation in young animals results in slowing down of growth rates. During slow wave or deep sleep a large amount of growth hormone is produced and this, in turn, stimulates protein synthesis and speeds up cell division and multiplication, both essential steps for growth and repair. This mechanism is well illustrated in athletes who engage in heavy exercise. They can be shown to get more slow wave sleep and to produce more growth hormone.

The energy charge of brain cells, which is related to the high energy phosphate content of the cells, can be calculated. Sleep deprivation results in a lowering of the energy charge while slow wave sleep brings about a rise and prepares the cell for action.

These findings help us to understand the connection between sleep and the processes of mental and physical restoration. They also suggest that increased stress demands increased sleep as is the case in athletes.

Patterns of Sleep and Sleep Needs

According to Nilse Webb the three-day-old infant will sleep almost seventeen hours per day; by six months this will have decreased to fourteen hours and gradually over the ensuing years our daily quota of sleep drops to below eight hours. At first sleep is taken irregularly. Then, between the ages of one and two the bulk of it is taken at night while some ten to fifteen per cent is taken during the day.

There is some misconception as to the amount of sleep required at different ages. Everyone agrees that the infant needs a lot of sleep – and gets it. The average adult requirement seems to be less than eight hours and it used to be thought that the very old need even less. An excellent study of actual sleep was carried out in 1968 by George S. Tune[4] who asked a large number of subjects to keep sleep charts for a period of eight weeks. The mean duration of sleep in the decade twenty to twenty-nine years was 7 hours 41 minutes. By the decade fifty to fifty-nine it had fallen to 7 hours 16 minutes. Thereafter it showed a rise to 7 hours 53 minutes in the sixties and 7 hours 40 minutes in the seventies. Night sleep was admittedly less in the aged but this was supplemented by cat naps during the day. It is interesting that the very old revert to the irregular sleeping patterns of the very young. Another unexpected finding was that women tended to sleep less than men. This work suggests that most adults will sleep less than the commonly recommended eight hours. However the discrepancy may be due to a confusion between hours spent in bed and hours asleep and it is quite possible that, although most people spend eight hours in bed, they will sleep only seven and a half hours or fractionally more or less. All this only tells us what people do and not what they should do and we may find that a little extra sleep is not only physiologically possible but indeed beneficial.

Nathaniel Kleitman believes that there is a Basic Rest Activity Cycle (BRAC) both in sleep and in wakefulness. In sleep, the pattern is fairly clear. Approximately one hour of non REM sleep is followed by twenty to thirty minutes of REM sleep making a total of about ninety minutes, which is repeated, with slight changes of the formula, several times a night. Non REM sleep can be regarded as the resting phase of the cycle and REM sleep as that of partial activity. Day-time BRAC is less obvious but if subjects are allowed to do as they please they will tend to break off all activity every ninety minutes or so and take a little rest or nibble at some food. The coffee break in so many offices and shop floors, occurring at 10.30 am, also divides the morning into ninety minute periods. A drowsiness after food or even a cat nap may similarly be an expression of the desire for inactivity in this cycle. Kleitman summarizes, 'There is a short term basic rest activity cycle in the functioning of the Central Nervous System of higher vertebrates that, although independent of the alteration of sleep and wakefulness, periodically modifies both these states.'

It may be that our Western way of life with its emphasis on productivity during the hours of daylight has forced us into a pattern of sleep which, although acceptable, is not in fact 'natural'. Perhaps the infant new from the womb knows better. Perhaps the people of the East who indulge in a siesta after the midday meal, have a more natural rhythm. An awkward question we should ask is whether our present sixteen hour day is the best possible arrangement, not only economically but physiologically and from the point of view of the preservation of good health? Could we possibly improve output and health by some other system? Should we learn from the animal world, the infant and the old and perhaps divide the sixteen hours cycle into two? It is certainly very tempting to those of us who are not so robust and tend to show signs of wear and tear when exposed to the accepted harsh routine. The proponents of a midday rest or sleep will have considerable opposition. Industrialists and business men will not approve. The energetic amongst us will think that society is going to the dogs, is becoming flabby and weakminded. Sleep researchers will point out that day-time sleep has a different quality about it and this is true. If sleep is taken during the day there will apparently be more of stage four sleep and less of REM sleep – but so what. Nowhere is it ordained that we should have exactly twenty-five per cent REM sleep whatever the circumstances.

It would not be right, however, at this stage, to advocate a universal change in sleeping habits. That would be premature and based on inadequate experience; but should we find, through future research, that mental and physical health benefits from an altered pattern of sleep, then a change will have to be seriously considered. For the present we would only suggest that those who find the pace of life too fast and stressful might consider a mid-day rest and those who have actually fallen ill through fatigue and strain waste no more time and snatch some added rest if at all possible.

Sleep and Illness

Doctors have advocated increased rest or sleep for a multitude of disorders from time immemorial. Often it was their only tool. It was as readily available as water and air and was not dependent on modern technology or chemistry. And rest, in an ill-defined way, still plays a prominent role in our therapeutic armamentarium. It is advocated for a wide range of ailments both chronic and acute. Examples of the former might be tuberculosis or rheumatoid arthritis; of the latter pneumonia, ulcerative colitis, coronary thrombosis and severe mental breakdown.

When prescribing rest there are many doubts and uncertainties in the physician's mind. Is the issue solely of more rest or is it one of sleep? In general it may be said that where the general health of the patient is good and a part only of his body is affected by injury, inflammation or impaired function, then rest alone is needed. But where the local disease has resulted in constitutional malaise or where, by improving the reparative processes of the whole body, the local disease may be improved, extra sleep as opposed to merely rest is required. Should added rest or sleep be given for a limited time only or should at least part of the extra quota be continued indefinitely? The common-sense answer to this must be that if the disease is one which may drone on, aggravated by stress and insomnia then there is good reason for a prolonged higher ration of sleep. What reservations and fears should we have about added rest and sleep? These measures cannot be undertaken lightly. Past experience has taught us that there are many pitfalls which are ignored at our peril. Excessive rest can lead to disuse atrophy or wasting of muscles, to loss of bone calcium from the skeletal system, to the formation of calcium stones in the renal tract, to the stiffening or even fixation of joints. Blood clots can form in veins through which the flow has become too sluggish because the muscles are not pumping blood through them, as they do in exercise, and some of the clots can become detached to lodge in a major blood vessel in the lungs. Excessive rest in the elderly can rob them of initiative and make them prematurely dull mentally, and passive physically. Deep sleep induced by heavy sedation may also interfere with normal body movements in sleep, especially in the old, and bring on pressure ulcers over bony points. So, for all these reasons, we must prescribe sleep and rest intelligently, always taking care to ensure adequate exercise of body and mind, and adequate movement of joints, between rest periods. Sleep has intrinsic value but, in addition, it is a means of priming the mind and body for healthy activity which is equally essential.

Sleep is linked to disease in a dynamic manner. It will not only influence the latter but be influenced by it. In other words there is a two-way traffic. We are beginning to understand how sleep as a whole, and its various stages, influences some diseases. We can observe the influence of mental disease, for example depression or schizophrenia, on sleep and we can see how physical conditions such as pain, fever and shortness of breath will affect sleep.

Patients with specific diseases in which the quality of sleep was suspected to play a part, have been carefully investigated in sleep laboratories. Armstrong found that, almost without exception, the duodenal ulcer sufferer showed tall peaks of gastric acid production coinciding with bouts of REM sleep. Similarly, Nowlin demonstrated that the cardiac patient who experienced nocturnal attacks of anginal chest pain was found to suffer pain more commonly some five to ten minutes after a REM phase. However no association was found between asthma and the various phases of sleep. Low blood cortisol in the early hours of the night might easily be partly responsible for nocturnal asthma. One would not expect REM sleep with its transient rise of blood cortisol to aggravate wheezing, it would indeed tend to counteract it.

Looking at these findings, particularly in the case of the ulcer patient, one might be tempted to manipulate sleep to eliminate the harmful phases. It would, however, be a retrograde step to use barbiturates in order to do this. In any case the acid peaks of the peptic ulcer patient can be dealt with quite satisfactorily by the use of anti-cholinergic drugs which inhibit acid secretion. Nevertheless this aspect of research is fascinating and offers hope of influencing disease by altering the quality and quantity of sleep.

Sleep disturbances in mental disease have been extensively studied. We need to refer here only briefly to two common mental diseases – depression and schizophrenia. In the former we often find a low arousal threshold, possibly the result of a high level of anxiety, accompanied by frequent awakenings and especially early morning waking. The dream content is likely to be unpleasant, if not frightening and if it should become intolerable it will cause wakefulness. There seems to be little stage four or deep sleep. In the manic phase of depression REM sleep is decreased while in the depressed phase it is increased.

In our view there is a link between chronic fatigue and some forms of depression. The high level of anxiety which is so often present in these patients leads to over-stimulation of brain cells, disturbed sleep and brain cell exhaustion. There follows decreased mental efficiency, and, by virtue of poor stimulation of the pituitary-adrenal axis, general body fatigue and physical inefficiency. This leads to lack of self-confidence, low self-esteem and depression. The feeling of inability to cope produces more anxiety and so a vicious circle is set up.

A recent publication lends support to this view. Doctors G. Allen German and H. G. Stampfer, writing in *The Lancet*[5] divided a group of depressed patients into two categories. The first, nineteen in number, suffered from a primary depressive disorder, the second, eight in number, had become depressed as a result of disagreeable and stressful life events. The latter also experienced considerable exhaustion. A single injection of a powerful new hormone (Hypothalmic releasing factor) was given to all the patients but only the second category responded. After a prolonged and natural sleep they recovered their energy and drive and dramatically lost their depression for a period of several months. The authors concluded that the new hormone 'can be strikingly effective in certain types of depression, especially where prolonged stress and exhaustion have played a role.'

The schizophrenic usually suffers from disorganized sleep, the onset of which is often delayed. There are frequent periods of wakefulness perhaps brought about by hallucinations, perhaps by anxiety-laden dreams. If REM sleep is inhibited then a rebound increase, as would occur in the normal subject, does not take place. The significance of this finding is not clear.

Another interesting by-product of work on sleep has been an increased understanding of such conditions as sleep walking, sleep talking, narcolepsy (brief bouts of involuntary sleep during the day) and sleep paralysis. From what has been said on body function in REM and non REM phases of sleep it becomes apparent that all disturbances of sleep in which there is a loss of muscle tone must be related to the malfunction of REM sleep and all those disturbances in which tone and muscle function are maintained must be related to the malfunction of non REM sleep. Narcolepsy and sleep paralysis must therefore be placed in the former group and sleep walking and sleep talking in the latter. In sleep paralysis the patient wakes to find himself momentarily paralysed – which can be rather terrifying. Both these disorders can be helped by drugs which abolish or reduce REM activity. The dangers of sleep walking are well known, while sleep talking is just a nuisance. Drugs do not seem to be effective in these last two conditions. The parents of a sleep walker should ensure that doors and windows leading to danger should be locked and that harmful objects should be removed. They should not be too worried as the condition usually subsides spontaneously.

Insomnia

For our purpose, in the context of stress and fatigue, the most important aspect of sleep is an insufficiency of it, or, in other words, insomnia. It appears that, in this country, some fifteen per cent of men and twenty-five per cent of women regularly take hypnotics after the age of forty-five. This vast consumption of potentially toxic material has many unpleasant implications. It is a poor comment on the quality of our lives in modern society. It must signify a considerable measure of discontent, anxiety and fear. It must surely mean a lack of understanding of how to lead a normal, healthy, natural life. The availability of dangerous hypnotic drugs is linked with a high suicide rate, now fortunately diminishing as barbiturates are being replaced by less harmful hypnotics. It places an unnecessary economic burden on society and in the end, however hard we try, pharmacologically induced sleep does not give us the quality of natural sleep. For all these reasons it is vital to understand insomnia and attempt a cure, if possible, by natural means.

Lawrence Monroe has compared good sleepers with bad sleepers. In general the characteristics of the latter are: they exhibit more body movements per hour during sleep; they are at a higher level of physical arousal, being more easily disturbed by minor stimuli; they sleep for a smaller proportion of the time spent in bed; by use of a personality profile (the Minnesota multiple personality inventory), they are shown to have more neurotic traits than normal, ie more evidence of anxiety, depression and so on; and finally they are found by EEG observation to spend less time in REM sleep. It is difficult to decide, however, whether some of these abnormalities are the cause of insomnia or its effects.

The severity of insomnia should be judged not solely by decrease in time asleep but also by the quality of sleep. A subject might have too little REM sleep, he might be persecuted by nightmares or he may sleep the artificial, drug-induced sleep, and wake with feelings of drowsiness, confusion or headache.

A host of drugs will affect both the quantity and quality of sleep. First let us look at those which have an adverse effect and which should therefore be avoided unless there are overriding considerations for their use. The stimulants are perhaps the most undesirable. Amphetamine was at one time considered to be an antidepressant and, in combination with a barbiturate, the notorious 'Purple Heart' pill, was frequently prescribed. It has now been almost totally given up because of the high incidence of addiction. Its adverse effects are that it will impede sleep, increase the number of body movements and wake periods when sleep finally comes and delay the onset of REM sleep. Ritalin (Methyl phenidate), a mild stimulant, has likewise been found to be addictive and suppress REM sleep. Tenuate (Diethylproprion), which is used for slimming, decreases REM sleep and, together with similar compounds, is rarely advisable. Ponderax (Fenfluramine), another slimming preparation, does not decrease REM sleep but encourages a shift towards light, stage one sleep without increasing the number of awakenings. So, here too, there is not an entirely natural sleep.

If Amphetamine and related drugs are withdrawn after a prolonged period of use, then there will be a rebound phenomenon with early onset of REM and increased REM sleep, and these abnormalities may persist for up to two months. In addition anxiety, tension and fatigue are again experienced.

The barbiturates have little to recommend them. This group contains such drugs as Sodium amytal (sodium amylobarbitone), phenobarbitone, Soneryl (buto barbitone), Tuinal (a combination of Quinalbarbitone and amylobarbitone), Seconal (Quinalbarbitone) and many others. They are not identical, some having a rapid onset and short duration of action, others a slow onset and prolonged action, but they have in common the property of suppressing REM sleep. Ian Oswald had this to say about them – 'Gradually as tolerance develops their effect is lost. If the drug is then withdrawn, anxiety rises sharply, sleep is broken, is subjectively unsatisfying, and is frequently accompanied by nightmares.'

Addiction to amphetamines and barbiturates can now be better understood. Withdrawal leads to anxiety, insomnia, nightmares and general wretchedness; these effects are often suppressed by a return to the drug. The patient fails to realize that the symptoms were self-induced and due to withdrawal, instead he ascribes them to the unfriendly and hostile environment and to his state of stress and neurosis.

So it seems that a rapid escape from reality by the use of drugs is bought at a considerable cost – that of addiction and dependence.

The question might be asked – where do the antidepressants stand in all this? Are they safe or are they too addictive? There are two main groups. Drugs such as Marplan or Nardil, inhibit an enzyme that would destroy serotonin, thus increasing the available brain serotonin; and the tricyclic antidepressants, such as Tofranil and Aventyl, which increase the effectiveness of available serotonin. The former group is not so widely prescribed as the latter because their use involves unwelcome dietary restrictions.

Some members of both groups will aid sleep, others seem to decrease sleep requirements, while some actually impair sleep. They all interfere, in some measure, with REM sleep. One might therefore suspect a possibility of REM rebound and addiction. But this does not seem to be the case. Early experiments tended to show an absence of REM rebound. Later it was recognized that rebound usually took place but was often delayed. In spite of this, the antidepressants do not carry the risk of addiction and can easily be withdrawn after a period of use. Because some are more sedative and some more stimulant they are chosen with care and tailored to the individual needs of the patient. The more sedative can be given at night, while the more stimulant by day only.

There are some harmless hypnotics which do not affect REM sleep and are not addictive. In this group we find chloral hydrate and similar preparations such as Welldorm (dichloral phenazone), Mogadon (nitrazepam), and Tricloryl (triclofos). They are not very popular as they do not invariably succeed in overcoming insomnia. But, as they are safe, the doctor must risk his own popularity and insist on this mild type of hypnotic.

This review of hypnotics is by no means exhaustive but it has been made to distinguish between groups of drugs which could be addictive and those that are not. It is an important part of a doctor's duty, and perhaps of the patient's duty to himself, that disease should not be brought about by medication. That, after all, is self-defeating or worse.

Alcohol has been used as a nightcap and perhaps, in small quantities, it could be regarded as such, but it is not really to be recommended as it too inhibits REM sleep and may therefore bring about withdrawal symptoms including heightened anxiety, nightmares and insomnia. This in turn may persuade the subject that he needs more alcohol and so the cycle of addiction is started.

Theoretically there could be another reason why drugs causing REM suppression should be avoided. It is during the REM phase of sleep that some of the night's cortisol is produced. Barbiturates, Doriden and other such drugs are known to cause a decreased output of this hormone and so it could be argued that the subject will be less ready to face the world after sleep under their influence.

This chapter has been lengthy, yet many will say that the subject is so important that the opposite criticism could be made of it – that these pages have been sketchy and inadequate. We have had to steer between the scylla of insufficiency and the charybdis of boredom. So what is the right answer to the management of insomnia? It should be a common sense one, based on knowledge and understanding. To brush insomnia aside would be as fatal as to overrate its importance. We do not yet have an adequate yardstick for measuring sleep requirements. Our sleep needs may be no more than those that we are currently getting; remember that we have already looked at the varying sleep habits of children and adults. On the other hand there is the suspicion that we should be getting a little more sleep than we allow ourselves. Health is not just an absence of disease. It is a state of positive well-being and of high resistance to threatened illness. Our thesis has been that chronic fatigue plays a prominent role in the genesis of disease. On that basis we should try to be fully, not just partly, rested. Then we can be at our best and give of our best. The positive advantages of adequate sleep would be – a sense of well-being, a freedom from many physical illnesses that could, and do, beset us, an efficiency of the mind which includes alertness, a sharp memory and a capacity to withstand mental strain. And, in addition, a decreased proneness to anxiety and depression and an improvement in mental and physical output which would be a joy to oneself and a source of satisfaction to the community.

If we are convinced of the value of sleep, how do we set about getting it? Remembering the sleep-wake balance, we would, by natural means, try to tip it in favour of sleep when the right moment comes. There is no better means of bringing sleep about than healthy evening fatigue. Physical exercise, whether in sport, factory or field seldom fails to bring sound sleep. Mental exercise is almost as good and those who have difficulty in getting off to sleep might try a non-emotive task, involving concentration, before shutting their eyes, perhaps reading some serious literature, biography, or history, but not a thriller, pornographic paperback or income tax returns. A glass of warm milk or a hot bath are often helpful.

If we have behaved in an exemplary way and still cannot find sleep then the mind should be consciously freed from its anxieties, and the body purposefully relaxed. Why not set aside the failures and problems of the day and focus attention instead on pleasant experiences, past or future. If our troubles will not recede into the background we can try any number of mental exercises to displace them. Counting sheep might be useful if only one could visualize that animal. Some people find that constructing words or shapes out of logs is easier, or one might recite a poem to oneself or indulge in some kind of simple addition or multiplication. The essential thing is to chase away the anxiety creating problem.

Physical relaxation is increasingly being practised. One way would be to start at the tip of each finger or toe consciously relaxing the digit then moving up gradually along the limb to reach shoulder and hip. Then the rest of the body, particularly the eyes, facial muscles, neck, chest and abdomen are encouraged to be flaccid until the entire frame is comfortably limp – almost asleep. As each part of the body relaxes so one might feel a tingling sensation and an increased warmth in it. It is a self-hypnotic exercise, usually successful, which greatly helps the mind to relax as well as the body. By concentrating on giving instructions to parts of one's body one gains an unexpected bonus – the suppression or non-emergence of unwanted thoughts. Autogenic training is a particularly useful form of relaxation. If we wake during the night our problems tend to intrude again and bring about prolonged wakefulness. Here the remedy seems to lie in trying to continue the narrative of the interrupted dream, provided that it has not been a frightening one, and, in so doing, sleep returns.

If a patient, previously a good sleeper, finds he cannot sleep then, in the majority of cases, a crisis of sorts has developed, mild or severe, which must be dealt with. The problem should be unearthed, faced and solved wherever possible. In these circumstances it would be in order to tide the patient over his period of crisis and to give, for a short time only, a non-addictive hypnotic or tranquillizer. Some patients, in whom a depression coexists, will perhaps respond better to a sedative antidepressant given at night. If the hypnotic on its own does not produce a satisfactory result, then a tranquillizer or antidepressant can be added. By these means the majority of insomnias can be cured without recourse to harmful drugs. It is at this point that the doctor should be firm and not embark on an easier but far more dangerous course, that of the barbiturates. In some instances pain will impede sleep and this is not too difficult a problem as there are many potent analgesics and antirheumatic preparations which are effective, harmless and non-addictive.

It must be admitted that there are some crises which are never ending and some patients chronically neurotic, vulnerable and sensitive. In our opinion we cannot be too rigid with these cases and must make life tolerable for them by allowing them to continue on maintenance treatment with mild tranquillizers and hypnotics, keeping them under review in the rare event that their life circumstances should improve and permit treatment to be phased out.

Where the confirmed barbiturate addict, now fortunately rare, comes to a doctor he will want to assess the patient to see if there is a chance of weaning him off the drug. A careful explanation of the harmful effects of the particular addiction, of the benefits of substituting a milder drug, of the difficulties encountered during the period of withdrawal, and how to overcome them, will brief the patient and often motivate him towards co-operation. The offending drug is given in slowly reduced doses so that withdrawal symptoms are minimized. A more satisfactory drug (one which does not interfere with REM sleep) is given, at first in addition to the barbiturate, then on its own. During the period of withdrawal a regime of adequate exercise is encouraged. Given sympathetic handling many addicts can be switched to safe drugs. We are not, however, talking of hard drugs of addiction such as heroin – these present a more difficult problem and are, in any case, in the hands of the addiction clinics. It would of course be better to avoid use of harmful drugs in the first instance than having to treat the addict at all.

Thanks to the work of numerous scientists and doctors we now understand the nature of sleep better than ever before and we have learnt to respect the particular quality of sleep in all its phases. We no longer ask just for sleep but for natural, revitalizing sleep – REM and all, by means which will not harm us or impair some other function of body or brain.

At the risk of being accused of moralizing we must end this chapter on a slightly different note. Could it be that one of the main factors in inducing healthy sleep is a feeling of satisfaction, of contentedness, of achievement, of work well done, of having made a contribution to our family and the society in general and having earned the approval of those around us?

11

*

The Emotions

IF WE ARE RIGHT in blaming adverse psychological factors and disagreeable emotions for an important segment of disease should we not search for the culprits, examine them carefully in the light of day and render them as impotent and harmless as possible? This proposition, let us admit immediately, is impossibly grand and over-ambitious. It would require an immense study of all the grievances and injustices in the interaction between human beings and the creation of a utopian social order for which none of us has the qualifications. Yet we need not go to the other extreme of total inactivity. Let us for the moment limit our field and focus down on human emotions, on their meaning and definitions, on how they are generated and how they might be controlled when they can be shown to exert an evil effect. Our intention then is not to study all the psychosocial stimuli which are brought to bear on a human being and all the interactions between the individual and those that surround him, but to consider broad categories of such stimuli and their effect on emotional response and adaptation.

Stimuli impinging on a subject in the course of his daily activity may produce a neutral emotional response, a response of pleasure and satisfaction or one of displeasure and aversion. Neutral emotion is probably a contradiction in terms. If no emotion is generated it is not neutral, it is just not there. As an example one might cite a dull, repetitive action on a conveyor belt. It may give us no satisfaction, yet no dissatisfaction. There appears to be an indifference. The spectrum of emotion ranges then from fear, panic, anger and hate on the one hand through to a neutral or, perhaps, non-reactive zone to intense pleasure and ecstasy on the other with lesser emotions ranged in between. We cannot effectively discuss the role of emotions in human behaviour and their relevance to illness without a pause for some definitions. There is a constant inflow of stimuli, first through the main sense organs serving vision, hearing, taste and smell, touch and other skin sensations; then a host of sensations from the body organs and muscles and finally images and fantasies of all kinds which occur spontaneously, in the brain even when we are shielded from outside stimuli. Some stimuli do not reach consciousness. For example we may not be aware of sensations from our organs but nevertheless there will be an appropriate autonomic response to maintain a stable internal environment. Nor may we be aware of each stimulus from our muscles as we walk or play. Adjustments are made automatically by the spinal cord and cerebellum (the organ of co-ordination and balance). Similarly a stream of impressions reaching us through our ears and eyes, as for example, when we are driving, may be sufficiently noticed to direct us and keep us out of harm's way but may not be registered in our memory or evoke any emotion. Nevertheless a considerable portion of incoming sensations is associated with feeling states. Some of these may have an intrinsic value to the subject, others may set up drives to direct further action. A poem or a piece of music may produce approval and pleasure but demand no reaction. An approaching dog may induce fear or pleasure, and set in train flight or fondling. It is through perception of incoming sensations that we form an assessment and bring about the appropriate affective state. Perception then is a mental mechanism for weighing up incoming sensations, combining the different strands of sensations into a meaningful whole and, by comparison with previous experience, allowing a judgement to be made on the likely impact on ourselves.

There is some confusion between an affect and an emotion so it is just as well to differentiate between these words. An affect may be taken to be a disposition of the mind, a state of feeling, a general assessment of a complex of ideas which forms the kernel of an emotional state. In other words the mental portion of emotions. Finally we come to emotion itself. It has been defined as an agitation of the mind, a moving of the feelings, but this is an insufficient description, for the mind cannot be dissociated from the body and so it should include the visceral accompaniment of affect – the pounding of the heart, the sweating palms, the overactive gut and whatever physical response is evoked by a particular effect. Richard S. Lazarus[1] elaborates this concept further. He rightly points out that there are three components of the emotional response – the cognitive subjective (what we have called the perceptive part), the physiological (heart, gut response etc.) and the motor behavioural, the last referring to laughter, tears, grimaces, threatening or friendly behaviour etc.

In spite of enormous research efforts our knowledge of the anatomy and chemistry of the emotions is still limited but nevertheless it would be helpful to touch on these aspects of the subject to show that some conclusions can be based on tangible research findings and not merely on speculation and guess work.

Before the invention of the microscope it was just not possible to make anatomical sense out of the brain and its ramifications. Gradually it became clear that the cortex, the grey convoluted outer layer, was comprised of myriads of cells and that the inner white matter consisted of sheets of nerve fibres which either emanated from these cells and carried messages away from the cortex or belonged to cells in the spinal cord, or cell groups in the interior of the brain, and carried impulses towards the cortex. The messages which are carried to and fro are, of course, not specific and different according to the sense organ or group of cells from which they come but are all simple electrical impulses which travel along a central axon or cable, reinforced as they go by a conversion of chemical to electrical energy at the non-insulated portions of the cables. The speed of the electrical impulse is far slower than that along a strip, say, of copper wire, but nevertheless exceedingly rapid. Specific messages are converted into electrical impulses at the sensory end organs and these, on arrival at their destination, are decoded back to the original message.

The brain can be subdivided into hind-brain, mid-brain and fore-brain, and in the human being, the fore-brain has become a vast organ, far outstripping in size and complexity that of any other mammal. Yet the secret of the emotions is not to be found in this newly-acquired intellectual tool but in the older part of the fore-brain, which we have in common with other animals, the limbic system. After all it is clear that all advanced mammals including cats, dogs and monkeys have basic emotional responses in common with us. So we would expect the emotions to be located in the old part of the cortex, the mid-brain and the hind-brain. There has not, however, been a total standstill in the evolutionary process relating to these older parts and they have become more complex and refined in the course of time. We are then not totally identical with our animal friends on the emotional plane, but basic similarities remain and may well explain our behaviour when this escapes from intellectual control.

Before going on to describe some parts of the limbic system we should briefly reconsider the reticular formation which has already been described in the chapter on sleep. It lies in the strategic central portion of the hind-brain and mid-brain and then spreads, in a Y-shaped manner, into the thalamic masses of both hemispheres. G. Moruzzi and H. W. Magoun[2] have claimed that the reticular formation is essential to consciousness. It is the activating organ, described by one Scottish anatomist as 'a great court of criminal appeal.' When it is calm we sleep, when busy with incoming sensations it demands activity, giving priority where required. It can focus attention on particular fields of sensation and plays its vital role on memory and motivation. It has intimate links with the limbic system.

J. R. Smythies[3] gives a fascinating and wide-ranging account of our knowledge of the structure and behavioural function of the brain. With a quiet dig at the psychiatrist he says 'it would seem desirable that psychiatrists should have a close understanding of our present knowledge of the cerebral basis of emotion, memory, mentation and behaviour.' Probably the rest of us would also gain by a rudimentary knowledge of these matters.

In the last twenty to thirty years it has become appreciated that various groups of cells at the base of the brain play an essential role in emotion and even higher cerebral functions. The limbic system is a term which has been applied to a group of structures belonging to the older fore-brain and subserving emotion and some aspects of memory. There is little point in giving a detailed anatomical account of this system for a number of reasons. Its complexity is well nigh overwhelming and had better be left to neuroanatomists; the links between its various parts and more distant structures are not entirely clear cut and its functions are not that well determined that we can be dogmatic; and then, why should we overburden ourselves with facts unless these have a practical application. But we could look at one or two of the more dramatic parts of the system and talk about their functions, of which some are fairly well understood and some remain speculative.

As long ago as 1937 James W. Papez[4] suggested that there was a circuit of structures and connections in the limbic system concerned with the higher elaboration of emotion. The name limbic, by the way, comes from the Latin limbus or border and conjures up in the mind an area between the higher cortical centres and the vegetative areas of the brain. The limbic system looks a bit like a race course with broad sweeps of communicating fibres linking cell groups. Messages flow round this circuit, being modified by stimuli from many different parts of the brain. Some are discarded as insignificant, others are intensified. Concepts are elaborated and compared with previous experience to generate the appropriate affect and motivation.

The Amygdala (Latin for walnut) are a collection of nerve cells in the white matter of the temporal lobe. The older part of the Amygdala deals with the sensation of smell. The newer part forms one of the important structures of the limbic system.

By stimulation and destruction of the Amygdala in animals, its functions are beginning to be understood. Its influence on movement and on the activity of our organs need not concern us. In the behavioural field, in which we are interested, it is concerned with the searching response allied to curiosity, with aggressive defensive reactions, perhaps with motivation through a positive reward centre and finally with the learning or forgetting of some conditioned responses.

Knowledge of the functions of the Amygdala has, on occasion, been of use in the clinical situation – for instance surgical removal of the Amygdala in children who are suffering from temporal lobe epilepsy, and are also aggressive and destructive, results in the majority becoming obedient and calm.[5] Not only is the epilepsy controlled but they also show good social adjustment. The same operation in aggressive, psychotic patients brings about a reduction in aggressive behaviour, but there is often a price to pay – some degree of mental deterioration.

Stimulation of certain groups of cells in the Amygdala of cats will produce a reaction of rage with spitting, hissing, baring of claws, while stimulation of nearby cells inhibits these self-same actions. So there seems to reside in this area an element of choice between flight and fight, between aggression and peaceful behaviour. This decision has often to be made in a split second on the basis of an assessment of incoming stimuli both from the outside and the inside and this portion of the limbic system seems to be the king pin in the process.

The Amygdala are involved in certain learning processes. For example dogs can be trained to associate a stimulus with avoidance. This will occur if the stimulus is followed closely by an electric shock and this type of reaction is called a conditioned avoidance response (CAR). Another stimulus, if succeeded by the offer of food, may be linked with approval. S. Butowski showed that removal of the Amygdala was followed by a loss of discrimination between those stimuli. In other words the operation resulted in the impairment of the ability to acquire the CAR or a rapid loss of a previously learned CAR.

In this vital sphere of decision between flight and fight, between acceptance and avoidance, the Amygdala not only have authority but also power, for they can stimulate the pituitary-adrenal axis to cope with the called for activity. This is well illustrated by an experiment in which a healthy animal is found to respond to the stress of immobilization by a twofold rise of plasms of cortisol in thirty minutes. If the Amygdala are destroyed the same rise will take four hours.

Still in the temporal lobe and right next to the Amygdala lies a longish area of the old cortex which must have reminded some anatomist of a sea-horse because it has been dubbed hippocampus. It was for long a neglected and poorly understood area of the brain thought to be mainly concerned with the sense of smell. We now know that it plays a significant role in laying down a permanent memory store. If the hippocampus is destroyed on both sides then immediate memory is not converted to long-term memory. Patients with damaged temporal lobes (including the hippocampus) can retain a memory such as the name of a person they have just met or the plot of a story they have just heard for a time but, if their attention is drawn to something else, this memory is lost.

Naturalists like Konrad Lorenz have shown how memories are imprinted in birds, at a relevant stage of their development. Geese will learn to follow a mother or mother figure and, if given a human substitute, will learn to accept that person as a mother and follow her. Bilateral removal of the hippocampus in birds results in a permanent loss of such imprinted behaviour. One might regard this type of behaviour as being similar to a conditioned reflex and the interesting thought occurs that, in converse to the situation when the hippocampus is removed, excessive activity of that centre might lead to overimprinting or the laying down of unwanted conditioned reflexes. It is curious how in some persons an accident, say in the underground, will give rise to a permanent phobia of all undergrounds, while in others the same accident is made light of and soon forgotten, leaving no trace of fear. Could this difference be due to a hippocampus working overtime?

The manner in which these functions of memory are lost is not quite clear. Some think that if the hippocampus is destroyed the ability to convert immediate memory to long term memory is lost, others consider that memory has been laid down but that recall of such memories is mediated by the hippocampus and cannot take place without it.

The hippocampus also plays a calming and discriminating role. It analyses incoming sensations to sort out the relevant from the irrelevant and so inhibits unwanted responses. In pursuance of this policy it has the ability to inhibit unwanted pituitary-adrenal activity.

Chemical Changes in the Brain

Anatomy and function, with which we have dealt so far, are mere descriptions of structures and their activities and will remain relatively incomprehensible unless chemistry is added to give flesh and blood to these bare concepts. The basic unit of the brain is the neurone, that is the brain cell with its axon and dendrites (tiny branches) and it can only be brought into action by chemical substances impinging upon it whether through the bloodstream or at the synapse (junction) with neighbouring cells or with the axons of distant cells. So if we wish to know what brings into play groups of brain cells we must sooner or later study the nature and effects of these chemical substances.

There are two separate problems related to the chemistry of emotion. The first concerns the nature of the chemical changes which initiate and accompany emotion in the brain itself and the second the chemical changes which result from the emotions both within the brain and in the body as a whole, and probably more is known about the latter.

As we consider the problem we must not mislead you – we have not yet reached that depth of knowledge which allows us to explain laughter and tears in chemical terms. We are familiar with some of the hormones which circulate in the blood and play around the roots and branches of the brain forest but we can be sure that there are many gaps in our knowledge and that innumerable substances are at work in this region of which we have as yet no inkling. So the picture we can try to paint is incomplete and far from satisfying; but the attempt must be made.

Perhaps the best way of approaching the subject of chemical changes within the brain which are related to emotion, is to highlight a few of the known facts rather than try to carry out the impossible task of presenting an integrated account.

In discussing the neurochemical aspects of brain function Smythies reports several interesting observations. Two Swedish scientists have demonstrated, by special staining methods, that some groups of neurones in the mid-brain, hind-brain and hypothalamus, contain noradrenaline and others serotonin. The long axons of these cells are widely distributed throughout the brain. A knowledge of the anatomical distribution of the cells and of the chemical properties of their contained hormones leads to the belief that they play a major part in arousal, wakefulness, sleep and the emotional states. It will, for example, be remembered that orthodox sleep is mediated by serotonin while REM sleep by noradrenaline.

Let us consider noradrenaline separately for a moment. One would expect it to be involved in the reaction to stress and indeed it has been found that noradrenaline turnover in the brain is increased when an animal is subjected to stress. However if the degree of stress is augmented or prolonged then the turnover rate falls pointing to exhaustion. Here we could have a clue as to the nature of the mental component of human fatigue. Does this not suggest that some groups of brain cells can become depleted of their hormone content, be it noradrenaline, serotonin or some other chemical, and then become inefficient or fatigued?

In the chapter on Cannon we referred to sham rage, that is rage not mediated by the higher centres and not directed at any particular opponent. Experimental work has shown that, in this condition, noradrenaline is widely released in the brain.

When a moderate dose of noradrenaline is injected into a particular portion of the hypothalamus of the rabbit it will make defensive responses. Paradoxically enough when the dose is increased the animal will fall asleep.

P.B.H. Poschel and F. W. Ninteman made use of the experimental technique of self-stimulation to discover more about the role of noradrenaline. In this procedure an electrode is placed into an area of the brain which gives rise to a pleasurable sensation when stimulated. The animal learns to stimulate the point itself by pressing a lever or carrying out some other convenient movement. When drugs which modified the action of noradrenaline were given the rate of self-stimulation was altered. For instance drugs which increase the activity of noradrenaline also increase self-stimulating rates and this could well explain the popularity of the now almost defunct 'purple heart' pill which contains amphetamine. On the other hand drugs which counteract noradrenaline, such as largactil, will slow down self-stimulating rates. It seems then that noradrenaline stimulates the reward system.

In this respect it is interesting to note that there is evidence to suggest that both caffeine and nicotine act indirectly on the brain via an intermediate compound, probably noradrenaline. Experiments in animals confirm that noradrenaline is released at 'pleasure centres' in the hypothalamus in response to nicotine.[6] As very little noradrenaline crosses the blood-brain barrier it seems likely that drinking coffee and smoking tobacco bring about a simultaneous release of this amine in the brain and at the periphery, that is to say at sympathetic nerve endings and in the adrenal medulla.

Further it seems that brain levels of noradrenaline play an important role in the regulation of mood. Drugs, such as reserpine, lower brain noradrenaline and can cause acute depression. Conversely, some enzyme inhibitors increase noradrenaline and can alleviate depression. In other words, an increase in brain noradrenaline might represent a final common pathway to pleasure.

To digress for a moment, could it be that cigarette advertisements, which depict situations of high excitement, achieve their stimulating effect by an increased release of noradrenaline? This pleasurable effect of noradrenaline in the brain may also explain 'Nesbitt's paradox'[7] which points to the contrast between the smoker's subjective impression that smoking relaxes him and objective evidence of increased sympathetic activity as reflected in the raised pulse rate, blood pressure and blood fats. Increased noradrenaline is associated with many of the virtues claimed for smoking, such as increased alertness, greater powers of concentration, and lowering of error rates[8] – while withdrawal of cigarettes can cause temporary impairment of psychomotor skills such as those involved in simulated driving.[9] On the other hand, inhibition by drugs of the effects of noradrenaline on the body does not affect the smoker's satisfaction which suggests that its effects on the brain are the more important reinforcers of this dangerous habit.

To sum up then we can say that brain noradrenaline is concerned with REM sleep, with arousal and with the ability to cope with stress, with the expression of rage and with priming of the reward system. No doubt it has many other duties.

Serotonin is a chemical of many parts. On the one hand it induces orthodox sleep, on the other it seems to be needed for healthy brain cell function and the maintenance of a state of dynamism and cheerfulness which chases away apathy, gloom and depression. At any rate the three main groups of drugs which are used to combat depression all act by making serotonin more available. The tricyclic antidepressants such as Tofranil block the renewed-uptake of serotonin and noradrenaline in the cleft between nerve cells and so prolong their action. Drugs like Nardil prevent the breakdown of serotonin and noradrenaline in the nerve cell and thus increase the store in the cell. Drugs of this second group are not so popular with the general practitioner or patient as, in order to prevent side effects, a large range of foods (for example cheese, wine and marmite), and important drugs including some effective painkillers and remedies against high blood pressure, have to be avoided. Finally there is L.Tryptophan, a precursor of serotonin which, if given by mouth, will likewise increase the amount of available serotonin. Although expensive it is of great help in some forms of depression.

There is then a common thread in our approach to the physical treatment of depression. We utilize drugs which enhance the activity of serotonin, and perhaps also that of noradrenaline; and this leads one to speculate that a possible physical mechanism in the onset of depression is a partial depletion of these amines in certain groups of brain cells. It is surprising how often anxiety is linked with depression and this strengthens the impression that there exists in these patients a low threshold of arousal coupled with raised anxiety and high output of emotional energy which results finally in depletion of serotonin and noradrenaline and a state of depression.

Far less is known about Acetyl Choline which is unstable and therefore difficult to trap and measure. It is the chemical released at the junction of neurones in the autonomic nervous system and at the nerve endings of the parasympathetic system and therefore in this latter task, mediates peaceful biological processes. It has an important but as yet ill-defined role, in the brain itself. It is probably concerned, as it is in the case of the autonomic nervous system, in the transmission of impulses across gaps between many brain cells, particularly in the cortex. Some of the limbic pathways are cholinergic, ie mediated by acetyl choline. Whereas the reward system, as pointed out above, is stimulated by noradrenaline it appears to be inhibited by cholinergic drugs. This suggests there is a balance between the adrenergic stimulus which is positive 'go' and the cholinergic stimulus which is, in this instance, inhibitory or 'no go'.

Sex hormones also influence emotion and behaviour. The docile nature of the eunuch is well recognized. Similarly, oestrogens (female hormones) given to men who would prefer to play a female role, not only changes their appearance but also their attitudes. Androgens (male hormones) given illegally to female athletes will improve performance and the aggressive drive. But strange and unexpected behaviour can result from injection of testosterone (a male hormone) into specific places in the rat brain. An injection in one spot can produce a mothering behaviour in the male rat! While into another spot, less surprisingly, increased sexual drive.[10]

There may be, hitherto unsuspected, chemical substances which influence emotion through memory. These two states cannot be separated from each other. There are some basic stimuli which have no need of memory and will produce stereotyped genetically controlled emotions. In this way pain gives rise to fear and a gentle caress to pleasure, but most emotions in our complicated lives are evoked by association of the experience with previous memory of an emotion, be it pleasant or unpleasant. Experiences, by reason of memory, carry a symbolic value. A harmless white mouse will give rise to pleasure in some and terror in others and our memory bank is responsible for this difference in emotional arousal. Chemical influences upon memory could therefore be of the utmost importance. The more we understand about faulty learning and encoding in memory, and the more we can do to correct it, chemically or otherwise, the more readily we will be able to encourage advantageous adaptive behaviour and the removal of unwanted and harmful behaviour patterns such as phobias and chronic anxiety states.

A most striking and unusual experiment upon memory is related by Lausch. This particular work was carried out by Georges Ungar of Texas on rodents, but its results cannot yet be put to use in the human field. Rats and mice prefer to forage and feed in the dark. Ungar made a group of rats dislike the dark by electric shock. When they had acquired a preference for light they were killed and an extract of their brains was prepared which in turn was injected into mice. Before injections these mice spent 130-140 seconds out of 180 seconds in the dark. Afterwards they spent only 50-60 seconds out of each 180 seconds in the dark. A chemical substance had changed their preference. It was appropriately called scotophobin (fear of the dark). Research has proceeded so far that it can be prepared synthetically. This type of research brings hope that memory and emotion will one day be therapeutically influenced by chemical means.

Our short review of chemicals which are active in the brain gives us a glimpse of the importance of the subject. As a matter of general principle we would all like to see our brains function spontaneously and efficiently and our moods fluctuate as circumstances demand without the outside influence of drugs. However, where 'natural' means malfunction or distortion of brain function, we should be thankful to chemists who have unravelled some of the mystery of brain chemistry and are helping to rectify these faults.

Chemical Changes in the Body

We must now look at the second problem, that of the widespread chemical changes occurring in the body in association with the emotions. These may be regarded as being both due to the emotions and part of the emotional state. 'Due to' because the emotions have brought into activity the autonomic nervous system and the hormone controlling system in the hypothalamus to regulate the internal environment, and 'part of' because, according to definition, the visceral and motor concomitants of emotional states are regarded as part of that state. Fear is not just mentally perceived but is also experienced by the heart pounding, the mouth dry of saliva and the palms wet with sweat.

One of the main rate-limiting steps in the synthesis of new scientific ideas is the development of methods for testing them. Nowhere is this more clearly seen than in the area of stress research, where increasingly sensitive and specific methods of chemical analysis have made it possible to dissect in great detail the complex pathways by which psyche and soma interact.

Bioassay methods based on physiological responses were used by Cannon in the studies he described in his classic monograph, *Bodily changes in pain, hunger, fear and rage*, published in 1929. In this publication, he reviewed the then known properties of the complete extract of the adrenal medulla, 'adrenin'. 'Adrenin' was later shown to contain more than four times as much adrenaline as noradrenaline. The actions of 'adrenin' which could be demonstrated in a wide variety of states of emotional arousal, were to accelerate the heart rate, increase the blood pressure and coagulability of the blood, dilate the bronchioles, and alter the distribution of blood in the body.

Only by distinguishing between the physiological and biochemical actions of adrenaline and those of noradrenaline, and by devising methods for their differential biochemical estimation, has it become possible to develop more detailed theories capable of explaining responses to emotion. Daniel H. Funkenstein[11] put forward an hypothesis that adrenaline release would be specifically associated with an anxious emotional state, whereas noradrenaline release would be associated with an aggressive emotional state. Although originally largely conjectural, this hypothesis has since been backed by a considerable body of evidence. He devised a simple formula on the basis of work carried out on artificially produced situations of anger and fear. The existence of noradrenaline was now well established and its properties were known to differ somewhat from those of adrenaline, but accurate measurements in blood and urine were still difficult. So Funkenstein made some fairly justifiable assumptions. He argued that, where, in his experimental subjects, a rise in blood pressure was not associated with a rise in pulse rate this signified noradrenaline response, while the reverse would signify an adrenaline response. Unfortunately he failed to confirm these assumptions by actual measurement of catecholamine output.

The self-confident subject when frustrated in a task, did not blame himself (how could he be wrong) but factors in his environment, so his anger was directed outwards and his physical reactions were compatible with noradrenaline release. In the adverse circumstances of the experiment his performance was relatively good. The introverted, shy, self-critical subject reacted differently. When things went wrong for him it was plain that he himself was to blame. His anger was directed inwards and was accompanied by anxiety and fear. The physiological response was one of adrenaline secretion. Performance was poor as his high anxiety level had interfered with efficiency. It was an attractive concept. Anger outwardly directed would give rise to a noradrenaline reaction and improved performance, while anger inwardly directed an adrenaline response and poor performance. It fitted in with the stereotyped behaviour of different species of animals. The lion, whose adrenal gland produced mainly noradrenaline, never stooped to flight, whereas the rabbit whose adrenal output was mainly adrenaline never aspired to aggression. Man, with his more evenly balanced production of adrenaline and noradrenaline had a greater choice. He could behave like lion or rabbit.

Fred Elmadjian and his fellow workers,[12] who studied the behaviour of the urinary catecholamines in a wide variety of active and passive participants in sports, as well as in neuropsychiatric patients undergoing psychotherapy, concluded that active, aggressive emotional displays were related to increased excretion of noradrenaline in association with normal excretion of adrenaline.

Some apparently conflicting work has been reported by Marianne Frankenhaeuser in Sweden.[13] In many ways her methods resembled Funkenstein's – such as the manipulation of the situation to bring about specific moods – but there is more subtle isolation of emotional components and actual measurement of urine adrenaline and noradrenaline output.

In one experiment she divided her subjects into two groups, the first being inactive and relaxed, the second inactive but purposely made tense in anticipation of the interview. Anticipation gave rise to a considerable increase in adrenaline output but little increase in that of noradrenaline. In another experiment she compared a group carrying out mental work under strain with a group which was inactive. In the former group the output of adrenaline rose but that of noradrenaline did not. This contrasts somewhat with the results in a group engaged in physical work on a bicycle ergometer. In this situation both the output of adrenaline and noradrenaline rose. From these and a whole battery of similar experiments Frankenhaeuser concluded that adrenaline secretion was related to the intensity of the emotional reaction but not its quality which depended upon cognitive and situational factors. Noradrenaline was likewise related to the intensity of emotion, but to a lesser extent. And here again there was no connection between the quality of emotion and noradrenaline output. Its rate of secretion was closely linked with the physical demands of the body.

These studies were all based on the output of stress amines in the urine. But a better and truer picture of sympathetic activity at any given moment can be gained by measurement of actual blood levels of these hormones. One of us (M.C.) was able to do this using special methods of sample preservation and highly sensitive techniques. In general, it was found that situations which induced active aggressive emotions, such as racing driving, driving in city traffic, and public speaking, caused predominantly an increase in plasma noradrenaline. By contrast, situations characterized mainly by passive anxiety, such as parachute jumping, airline flight, dental surgery, and rock climbing, provoked almost exclusively a rise in plasma adrenaline. Responses to both amines could largely be suppressed by beta-blockade. The effectiveness of small doses of drugs such as Trasicor, which can be used to block the action of these amines, in reducing anxiety symptoms could be accounted for by postulating that this treatment interrupts a self-perpetuating spiral in which anxiety leads to adrenaline secretion and the associated symptoms, for example palpitations, increase the anxiety still further.[14] This explanation also provides a chemical basis for the suggestion made by William James[15] that anxiety symptoms can reinforce anxiety.

As well as explaining some of the physiological and biochemical correlates of anxiety, plasma estimations can also furnish information on changes accompanying more pleasurable states. Physically stimulating conditions such as cold and exercise[16] increase circulating noradrenaline; so also do emotionally stimulating activities, such as driving, coffee drinking and smoking. As described earlier this is why we might become 'stress seekers'.

Valentina Myager,[17] a Russian contributor to the Stockholm Symposium on stress in 1970, reported some very relevant and interesting material on chemical responses to psychic trauma. She discussed not only specific emotions but groups of symptoms. Fear gave rise to an increased output of adrenaline. In anger and irritation the output of both adrenaline and noradrenaline rose. Grief and tears, which have so far not been mentioned, were associated with a fall of catecholamines.

In the chapter on fatigue we postulated a low evening blood cortisol. Dr Myager described a similar state of affairs in most neurotic patients. She found a low seventeen ketosteroid (corticosteroid end product) content in their urine suggesting fatigue and exhaustion of the adrenal. In situations of high emotional strain she noticed a high catecholamine output and a low seventeen ketosteroid one.

Looking back then on chemical changes accompanying emotional states we can begin to form a fairly accurate and comprehensive picture. In the brain itself various transmitters of information and stimulators of endocrine and motor activity are at work. Noradrenaline, serotonin and acetyl choline are each concerned with their particular network of brain cells, activating or inhibiting them. Specific emotions are generated, particular drives are set up depending on the balance of opposing forces. In the body however, we find that intense emotion brings about a rise of adrenaline and noradrenaline. If physical activity is called for there will be a more pronounced increase in noradrenaline output.

But a rise in catecholamines is not the only change in response to emotion. There is also an increase in cortico-steroid production and a rise in the level of free fatty acids and other fatty substances such as cholesterol. Later on we shall see that the thyroid gland becomes more active and thyroid hormone levels rise. In states of calm, tranquillity, boredom and perhaps grief these chemical changes can actually be reversed. Scores of other chemical processes will, of course, take place in emotional states but we have only highlighted the principal actors and those which might adversely affect our health.

When we come to a study of disturbed mental and physical health due to social and psychological factors, this glimpse of the chemistry of the emotions will be of great help.

12

*

Social and Work Stress

SINCE THE DAYS of the Industrial Revolution it has been obvious that working conditions in factories, offices and shops are related to health, and numerous Factory Acts and Public Health measures testify to this recognition. Women and children have been protected from unduly long hours and excessively hard labour. By and large the danger to health caused by noxious chemicals and by the many physical hazards of industry have been removed. And yet the suspicion remained that the health of the working population was still at risk by reason of many less concrete, less tangible factors such as the pace of work, mental and physical exhaustion and the anxieties and fears brought about by competition and status seeking. The development of Psychosomatic Medicine focused attention on possible psychological factors in illness but, at first, workers in this field concentrated on interpersonal relationships in the family. They appeared to be shy of entering the industrial sphere. We are not saying that industrial psychologists and doctors ignored psychological factors in industry altogether, but it seems they took only two important points into consideration. The first being the workers' general welfare and the second the level of production. The third and perhaps essential factor – that of actual illness brought about by working conditions – has, up to recently, been neglected. We must admit that as a result of studies of work efficiency in relation to mental and physical fatigue work breaks and shorter hours have been introduced without loss of production, but there has been little realization that actual illness such as heart disease or rheumatoid arthritis might be related to stressful working conditions.

There were considerable difficulties in the path of the research worker. Not only was it hard to measure stress brought about by specific aspects of industry and to disentangle this from domestic stress and from personality factors, but the overall implications were frightening. There might have to be a major reappraisal of many of our industrial customs. Doubt might be cast on such matters as the length and grouping of working hours, on rotating shifts, on the conveyor belt system, on standards of safety and comfort and on the present turbulent state of industrial relations, and there might be an upsurge of litigation in the field of compensation. People would be inclined to blame their conditions of work for their every illness. Without knowledge, commonsense and restraint it could be an explosive and uncontrollable situation. Yet no disruptive and harmful consequences are likely to arise as a result of the investigation of psychosocial factors in the causation of distress other than claims for increased pay to make up for occupational stress. One can only envisage increased health and productivity.

We now have a clearer idea of what is meant by stress and there are accepted measures such as levels of blood cortisol, adrenaline and noradrenaline which will indicate that any particular individual is undergoing stress. We have learnt to create artificial situations leading to stress which mime the industrial setting, or we can isolate an actual work process which is stressful. So we can pin-point the work situation which gives rise to stress and we can measure the degree of stress which has been produced by that situation. What is more difficult is to link stress with specific diseases and it is this last stumbling block which prevents us from being dogmatic. We can be pretty certain that industrial stress does lead to disease but proof by cast-iron statistical means eludes us, at present, in the majority of cases. There are a number of variables which influence the scene and which cannot be ignored such as age, sex, genetic endowment, habits relating to exercise, diet, alcohol, tobacco and temperament. How are we to tell what proportion of the blame for a particular disease, thought to be caused by industrial stress, is, actually due to it and what proportion falls on domestic and social factors. Epidemiological research on a wide scale will probably help. However there will always be an element of doubt and uncertainty in apportioning blame and whereas one may be sure in a large population that an industrial or social factor is responsible for a certain illness yet, in any individual case, no decision can be reached. For example, doctors might have, en masse, a higher incidence of coronary thrombosis than clergymen and this is probably related to their conditions of work, yet, in any one subject, personal factors may outweigh work factors. Or again coal miners may suffer, as a group, from more rheumatoid arthritis than bakers but occupation cannot be blamed with certainty for the disease in any individual miner or baker. It seems therefore that we will come to recognize that, in a broad sense, certain industries give rise to certain stress situations and groups of diseases and, in consequence, we will wish to reduce these stresses but we will not penalize industry for individual incidents of disease, except where a direct causal link is clear.

Body Reactions in Psychosocial Stress

In April 1970 a conference, sponsored jointly by the University of Uppsala and the World Health Organization was held in Stockholm on the subject of Society, Stress and Disease.[1] Distinguished contributors, including 'the Father of Stress' Hans Selye, came from all parts of the world and their published work showed that a determined effort had been made to penetrate the mists surrounding the subject and to lay the groundwork for future research in depth. The work of the conference itself and the fruition of the seeds it has sown will transform our attitudes and influence our approach to the organization of industry for the benefit of society for decades to come.

Aubrey R. Kagan and Lennart Levi[2] make an exceedingly useful review of the effects of the environment and psychosocial stimuli on health. They remind us that Cannon, in 1929, formulated the theory that the organism reacted to emergency states, including those elicited by psychosocial stimuli, with increased adrenal activity. It was not, however, till 1954 that Von Euler and Lundberg, using new techniques, were able to demonstrate increased urinary excretion of catecholamines in human beings under stress. Their subjects were air force pilots undergoing the stress of a flight situation. Since then many situations have been found to bring about bursts of sympatho-adrenomedullary activity. The psychosocial stimuli might be unpleasant or pleasant and include driving a car, sitting university examinations, awaiting participation in sporting events and watching both pleasant and unpleasant emotional films. Psychosocial stimuli of longer duration, as in industrial situations, are known to result in correspondingly prolonged sympathetic activity. On the other hand experimental stimuli evoking responses of calmness and equanimity lower catecholamine excretion significantly below control levels.

It is not just the adrenal medulla which is provoked into greater activity by psychosocial stimuli of all kinds but also the cortex and so we find that stimuli arising in stressful situations of the type described above will bring about a rise of blood cortisol while conversely situations giving rise to boredom or calm will actually bring about a fall of blood cortisol. The response of the adrenal cortex is slower than that of the medulla and its supportive role is more prolonged.

There is evidence that thyroid gland activity is influenced by psychosocial stimuli and that a number of stress inducing experiences, such as sitting examinations, prolonged exertion without adequate sleep and exposure to noise will cause excess production of thyroid hormone. This, in turn, acts on many organs in the body speeding up the turn-over of biochemical processes.

One could go on describing the multitudinous physiological reactions which are brought about in the body by psychosocial stimuli but this would only confuse us. We can well imagine that no single part of the body escapes from the effects of stress as the blood stream and nervous system act as highways which overcome isolation. So on to some concrete examples which we shall take mainly from the report on the Stockholm Conference of 1970.

First let us see what effect pleasant and unpleasant emotions have upon catecholamine production. In some interesting work carried out by Lennart Levi, twenty healthy female clerks were shown a different type of film on four successive evenings. First came a bland selection of natural scenery films produced by Norwegian Railways. They induced a feeling of calm and relaxation amounting in some instances to boredom. It is not surprising that the output of adrenaline and noradrenaline in the urine actually fell for the period of the film. Then came Stanley Kubrick's tragic film *Paths of Glory* which evoked feelings of anger and excitement. The output of adrenaline rose, but noradrenaline was hardly affected. On the following evening a viewing of *Charley's Aunt*, in which the predominant reaction was one of amusement and laughter, brought about a similar response. The last film on the menu was *The Mark of Satan* which induced feelings of excitement and fear accompanied by a rise both of adrenaline and noradrenaline excretion.

It is not difficult to imagine a more innocuous experiment. No laboratory animals, no inconvenience to the human participants, not even any needles seeking blood samples. All the charming clerks had to do was to look at films and pass three lots of urine. Yet the experiment was informative. Non-disturbing psychosocial stimuli brought about no adaptive stress reaction, while both unpleasant and pleasant stimuli which evoked intense emotions brought about adaptive responses involving a high output of adrenomedullary hormones.

If similar emotional responses had been triggered by real-life situations, by actual personal involvement in the threatening or exciting scene, we might expect a physical response and a discharge of energy. But in the artificial setting of modern society the experience is either vicarious and evokes no physical activity or, although relevant to ourselves, activity is suppressed because our culture demands inhibition of both physical and intellectual aggression. In this kind of situation the build-up of catecholamines might, and probably does, result in harmful biochemical changes inside the body.

A somewhat similar experiment was carried out using film material with a sexual content. About fifty members of each sex were exposed to these 'psychosocial' or should we say 'psychosexual' stimuli and the catecholamine output was measured before and after the film. The outcome was unexpected. Males excreted far more adrenaline and noradrenaline than females. Perhaps this is in keeping with male aggressiveness and female passivity in the sexual role or to male sensitivity to vision of beauty and female sensitivity to the gentle touch.

From this kind of experiment and the work of Holmes and Rahe, on life change and the Cluster theory of disease we learn that stress is not only a response to the threatening and unpleasant stimulus but may just as well develop from the more intense, pleasant stimulus. And this would be logical as the basic process is one of adaptation. We may feel that we do not need to adapt to pleasure – it is, after all, just what comes naturally – but the fact is being recognized that pleasant events require and must obviously need, the same kind of preparation as unpleasant ones. Of course our reserves of energy must become available at times of communal rejoicing be it a wedding, a dance or competitive sport. Pleasant experiences may be accompanied by tension, excitement, the need for quick thinking and physical preparedness. This situation is well represented graphically by Levi and his colleagues in the following diagram.

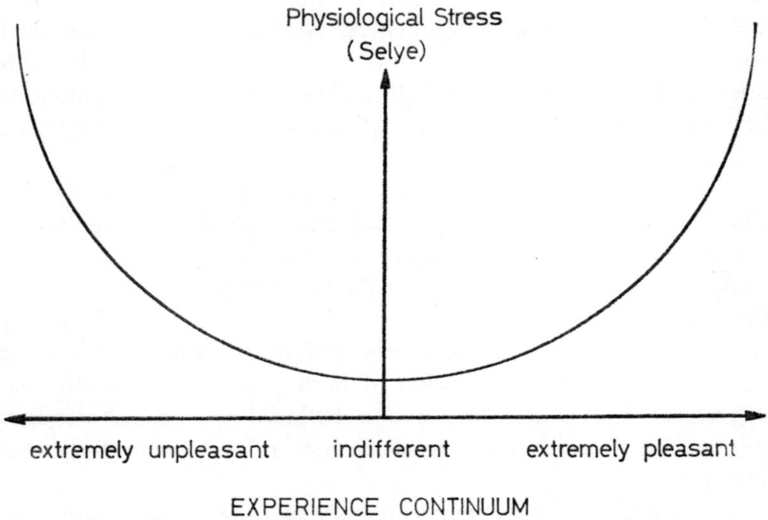

Fig XIII. Relationship of experience, both pleasant and unpleasant, to stress

The stress response is not by any means always harmful, especially if energy and various metabolites are used up in a healthy way. However we should not dodge the possibility that some pleasant experiences might be both stressful and harmful. This does not mean that we should avoid all harmful experiences. A totally sheltered and calm life might be harmless but at the same time it would be deadly dull and flat, and most of us are prepared to take some risks for the sake of a rich and varied life.

All we have shown so far is that various states of emotion are associated with increased catecholamine production and excretion. But that does not amount to disease. Is there any hard evidence that illness follows on specific social stress? This state of certainty has not been reached but evidence is accumulating and the following two pieces of research are highly suggestive and deserve careful study.

Lars Carlson, Levi and Oro[3] have shown that certain potentially harmful changes occur in a stress situation and that these threatening changes can be prevented. Thirty-three male volunteers were divided into three groups. The first group was made up of eleven men who acted as controls and remained sitting and idle. The other groups were engaged in a work project under conditions which provoked distress. One of these two groups was treated with nicotinic acid, a drug which is known to lower blood fat levels, for the week preceding the experiment; then, after a sixteen hour drug-free period, they were given nicotinic acid again for the first three hours of the experiment. The other group received no treatment. The men were observed for three two-hour periods during the second of which the two experimental groups were given stressful work which consisted of sorting out ball-bearings to the accompaniment of distracting noise and lights. One might think this was not very heavy work as far as the physical effort was concerned, but it was rendered difficult by the obstruction to clear thinking. The subjects in the work group betrayed their stress by a rise of pulse rate and blood pressure. Urinary output of noradrenaline and adrenaline increased appreciably. The untreated work group in addition showed a considerable rise in blood fats while the treated group developed no such response. Now high levels of blood lipids or fats, if maintained for prolonged periods, are suspected of causing arterial damage; so we can say that groups of people whose work leads to high blood fat levels are more at risk than those in whom no such response is evoked. We have, of course, not actually proved that disease has followed as a direct result of the work situation. The interesting point of this experiment lies in the fact that rises in blood fats can be anticipated and prevented by appropriate action. The effectiveness of nicotinic acid was well demonstrated in this experiment. This does not mean that we should stuff stressed business men and factory workers with this particular drug, as it happens to have some unwanted side effects such as flushing, but it does suggest that, in future, ways will be open to correcting the evil effects of stress by some innocuous means, and indeed there are other pharmacological candidates already in view which will protect against the sympathetic overdrive of the stress reaction such as β adrenergic blockers which will be discussed later.

Jan Froberg, and his fellow workers in 1969[4] used a group of senior Swedish army officers, whose average age was fifty-six, to test the effect of prolonged activity and sleep deprivation on body function. These men were asked to spend alternating three hour periods on a shooting range and military staff work for a total of seventy-five hours. No relaxation or sleep were allowed. Stimulants, smoking and walking were forbidden. The first period of three hours was used for the purpose of control. The results of the experiment were remarkable. Not only were these men physically and mentally exhausted, as would be natural at their age, but there were striking objective bodily changes. The red cell sedimentation rate, which is linked to the activity of inflammatory processes in the body, rose by thirty-eight per cent; protein-bound iodine, a measure of thyroid function, increased by nineteen per cent indicating greater metabolic activity or turnover; and serum iron decreased by twenty-six per cent. A similar experiment was conducted by Levi, in which he used a mixed bag of thirty-one younger army officers and corporals whose average age was twenty-nine. They were asked to perform exclusively on the shooting range, again for a total period of seventy-five hours, of which the first three hours served as a control period. Psychological, biochemical and electrocardiographic reactions were observed. Basal fatigue and distress were given a rating of one hundred and the subjects, who were questioned every three hours, were asked to report their fatigue and distress levels by reference to the percentage increase over basal levels. Distress ratings rose to one hundred and fifty per cent, fatigue ratings to as high as three hundred per cent, while efficiency, which was measured by the number of shots and the number of hits in a three hour period, fell correspondingly.

Urinary excretion of adrenaline followed a circadian pattern in spite of uninterrupted activity, and showed lowest levels after midnight and highest levels in the afternoon. There was a slight stepladder type of increase over the three days in the twenty-four hours catecholamine output. Efficiency was at its lowest and fatigue at its highest during the period of low catecholamine output. As in the other experiment the red cell sedimentation rate increased, by 168 per cent, protein bound iodine rose, by thirty per cent, and serum iron fell, by fifty-two per cent. In some twenty-five per cent of subjects the electrocardiogram (ECG) showed changes which suggested mild insufficiency of the blood supply, or mild damage of the heart muscle during the vigil, which were completely reversed to normal a day or two after the experiment.

Here then is evidence of clear bodily changes, of a potentially harmful kind, in a situation which mimics combat stress of real life. It must be pointed out again that none of the officers and men actually developed a permanent disease as a result of their imposed stress experience but, as the ECGs show, they were not far off such a condition and the inference is that if this kind of experience were maintained or often repeated real damage would take place.

Even more striking cardiac changes, brought about this time, by the stress of public speaking, were described by Peter Taggart, Malcolm Carruthers and Walter Somerville.[5] This team from Middlesex Hospital and St Mary's Hospital, London, made use of the situation where a lecturer confronts an audience. To anyone sitting in the auditorium the lecturer manages to convey the picture of a man who is knowledgeable, confident and at ease. Few will be aware of the actual state of affairs – of the anxiety amounting in some cases to panic which most public speakers feel, even when experienced and fully briefed on their subjects. Taggart and his co-workers were able to record unobtrusively a continuous electrocardiographic tracing by means of remote radio telemetry. These tracings revealed the cardiac turmoil which lay behind the calm exterior mask. Twenty-three of their subjects, mostly doctors, were considered to be normal, healthy persons. A further group of eight, all lay speakers, were known to suffer from coronary artery disease.

Using a double blind method 'Trasicor' (oxprenolol), a β adrenergic blocker, or a placebo was given to eight of the former group and all the members of the latter group one hour before lecturing. As its name implies, it blocks the action of catecholamines on the sympathetic nerve endings in the heart muscle and should therefore prevent a rise of pulse rate under emotional stress. Venous blood samples were taken a few minutes before and after speaking.

The results were dramatic. While the normal resting pulse is sixty to eighty per minute, the mean pulse rate in the normal group while speaking, was 151 per minute with a range of 125 to 180, and in the coronary group it was 133 with a range of 115 to 160. The effect of Trasicor was equally remarkable. It reduced the mean speaking pulse rate in the healthy group to eighty-seven and in the coronary group to seventy-seven.

When a subject suffering from coronary heart disease is made to exercise, the ECG shows changes which indicate deficient oxygenation of the heart muscle (typically ST Segment depression). This change developed in one of the twenty-three healthy subjects and in three of the coronary subjects while speaking. Emotional factors, leading to a rapid pulse, were thus able to bring about changes normally associated with physical exertion.. Trasicor dramatically and convincingly abolished these changes.

The normal rhythm of the heart is, by and large, regular showing only minor variations in rate with different phases of respiration. For reasons not fully understood extra or 'ectopic' beats or other abnormal rhythms may occur in healthy or diseased hearts usually in conditions of stress. In this experiment ectopic beats, of more than six per minute, occurred in six of the twenty-three healthy subjects and five of the seven coronary subjects while speaking. These too were abolished by Trasicor.

As we have learnt to expect in this kind of stress situation there was a rise of catecholamines, due in the main to noradrenaline and not adrenaline, in twenty-one of the twenty-three normal subjects. Blood fats in the shape of free fatty acids and triglycerides rose considerably, the former by some fifty per cent, the latter by about twenty-five per cent. Blood cholesterol levels remained unchanged, probably because of the timing of blood samples. Had blood been taken later a rise in cholesterol would also have been demonstrated. Having witnessed the remarkable effect of Trasicor on the pulse and heart it will be no surprise to learn that it also inhibited the rise of catecholamines and blood fats.

This research work has shown up public speaking for what it is – a highly stressful activity, arousing strong emotions and bringing about all the tell-tale evidence of stress – dramatically raised pulse, outpouring of catecholamines and subsequent rise of blood fats. We begin to appreciate the potential dangers of the situation with the heart being undoubtedly put at risk. This being lowest in young healthy, calm subjects and highest in the older, perhaps already coronary, more emotional subject. It is surprising that public speakers do not indeed fall ill more often; but from time to time we do hear of some distinguished person or other who has made one too many after dinner speech and who collapses at the table. Yet public speaking is unlikely to fall into disuse. Vanity and necessity will bring us to our feet, but perhaps a small pill one hour before speaking will lessen the risk. Certainly this work has shown that a β adrenergic blocker will suppress the racing pulse, the ectopic beat, the ischaemic ST Segment and the unwelcome rise of blood fats.

It might be argued that we do not have enough understanding of stress in Industry to permit major changes and we have to admit that hard statistics are often lacking, but we believe that enough is now known to allow a start to be made in laying down a few principles for action.

What then are the facts? We might approach this subject from two angles. First, what bearing has social class and sex on illness and survival? Second, what is the connection between specific occupations and specific diseases?

Population Studies

It might be a good plan to start with the excellent ten yearly review of occupational mortality by the Office of Population Censuses and Surveys, which was last carried out for the years 1970 to 1972 and published in early 1978.[6] The cold facts which emerge reflect the state of the nation more accurately and objectively than could any investigation by a whole team of newspaper and TV reporters. And the facts are not all comforting. Perhaps the welfare state has not had time to achieve its aims, perhaps it has set about it the wrong way. The disparity between the lives and fortunes of the rich and poor persists. Health and survival are still strongly related to social class and occupation.

The report emphasizes that there is a complex relationship between occupation and health. Factors intrinsic to the occupation will affect all its workers. They will share the same exposure to noxious dusts and chemicals. But each worker brings certain external factors to the work place. His particular personality, his attitudes, his own strengths and weaknesses. Then finally the income he derives from his work will to some extent determine his life style and the comforts or hardships he will experience.

A household survey contrasts the material possessions of the professional class and the unskilled labourer. Whereas both groups have lavatories and TV sets, perhaps the basics of civilized life, it is only the professional class that almost uniformly own telephones, central heating and refrigerators. These are scant in the ranks of the labourer.

In 1970 the previous five social classes were increased to six by subdividing social class III into two tiers namely, III N non-manual and III M manual, skilled occupations. That gives us now social class I – professional and similar occupations, II – intermediate between I and III, IV – semi-skilled and V – unskilled occupations.

The main index of comparison in the survey is the Standardized Mortality Ratio (SMR). This is a simple concept of the number of deaths observed in the group under study compared with the number of deaths expected in that group, taking into account the age and specific death rates in England and Wales, expressed as a percentage. Thus the SMR is: deaths observed, divided by deaths expected, multiplied by one hundred, and so a figure below one hundred is better than average and a figure above worse than average.

The unhappy fact is that the SMR for social class I is 77, while for social class V it is 137. Another indicator of this disparity is that men aged fifteen in social class I may expect to live $3\frac{3}{4}$ years longer than their fellows in social class V. There may be numerous reasons for this state of affairs but one of the saddest is that the greater the need for medical services the smaller the use that is made of them. This is well illustrated by advantage taken of dental and immunological services by children in the different social classes. Sixteen per cent of children in social class I had never visited a dentist. In social class V this figure was thirty-one per cent. Only one per cent of social class I children had not been inoculated against diptheria. In class V it was eleven per cent. In much the same way there is evidence that the unskilled worker takes little heed of health education campaigns aimed at a reduction of alcohol and tobacco consumption.

Mortality is affected not only by social class but also by region. Over the years the North West of England has been a black spot for health. For the whole of the last century the SMR in that part of the country has hovered between 110 and 119 while during this period the South West of England and East Anglia have enjoyed SMRs below 100 and even below 90. If we focus down on to specific occupations within the social classes and specific diseases the same regional variations are apparent. Workers in the electrical trades in the North West suffer from more coronary artery disease than those in East Anglia, the SMRs being respectively 152 and 88. Clerical workers are similarly disadvantaged when comparison is made between the North West and the South West of England, the respective SMRs being 142 and 106. It looks as if one must choose one's birthplace but if that is not possible, and it rarely is, then we should attempt to reproduce in the more hazardous parts of the country the amenities of the sheltered areas. Is the disparity due to pollution, to stress or to poverty? The answers to this problem and their remedies must be found.

A factor greatly influenced by changing attitudes in the last few decades is the proportion of women employed in Industry. In 1931 it was ten per cent, by 1951 it had increased to twenty-three per cent and in 1971 it had reached forty-four per cent. It used to be possible to assess the effects of occupation on mortality by comparing mortality rates of men who worked in Industry with those of their wives who by and large did domestic work only. This is becoming impossible. The health of increasing numbers of women will be affected by their occupations and they will have the same interest as men in bringing about sensible and healthy conditions of work. We have yet to learn what will be the cumulative effect on women of the stresses of childbirth, childrearing, domestic work and employment. Perhaps Women's Lib has overestimated women's ability to cope on equal terms. Perhaps they should, after all, be privileged by a shorter working day and hours of work more suitable to family life.

When mortality from a particular disease rises in step with the social classes I to V this is called a positive social class gradient and it is not surprising that there should be a positive gradient in all the infective and parasitic diseases, in the malignant diseases, in accidents, poisonings and violence and in the respiratory diseases. But strangely and almost inexplicably there are negative gradients. For example in 1930-32 the SMR for angina pectoris (chest pain related to exertion in disease of the coronary arteries) was 237 for class I falling to 67 for class V. But this advantage has been wiped out by time and the figures are now almost reversed. Another example is in relation to asthma. For this condition the SMR amongst boys in social class I is 176. In social class V it drops to 93. Here being a member of social class I is of positive disadvantage. Could it be that in the smaller families to be found in social class I the parent-child conflict, often at the root of asthma, is greater?

Arthritis and rheumatism are diseases which weigh heaviest on the least privileged. For every sufferer in social class I and II there are at least four among partly-skilled and unskilled workers, social classes IV and V.[7] The magnitude of the problem can be judged by the number of working days lost and the number of people disabled by these conditions. In 1970, thirty-seven million working days were lost in Britain or nearly twelve per cent of the total time lost through all illness. Of 343,000 people registered as handicapped by local authorities in 1972, twenty-five per cent suffered from rheumatism.

One can readily appreciate that hard physical work under cramped conditions leads to an additional amount of rheumatism and joint disorder. For example we get prolapsed discs in floor moulders working in iron foundries and we find arthritis in exposed joints in coal miners and dockers.

If we accept the conclusion reached in the chapter on chronic fatigue we will recognize an element of work exhaustion in the development of the rheumatic disorders. The less affluent will have less equipment to reduce home chores, will obviously not engage domestic help, will manage larger families and, in general, will have more cause for fatigue through long hours of physical work both at factory and home. This is not yet brought out by official surveys but may well have a bearing on the preponderance of the rheumatic disorders in social classes IV and V.

Within a social class mortality might differ. Ischaemic heart disease (where coronary blood vessels are narrowed) is more prevalent among employers in social class II than among managers. The burden of being an employer seems to heighten the risk.

There is a positive, adverse, relationship between social class and disease mortality in many other fields. In mental disorders we have a gradient from 59 to 87 in the non-manual groups and from 55 to 286 in the manual. The same picture is seen with regard to ulcers of the stomach and duodenum. Suicide is strikingly related to social class particularly among manual groups where the gradient rises from 77 in III M to 184 in V. These figures speak for themselves and need no horrific adjectives to bring the point home.

Over the years a social class gradient may be reversed. If we take hypertensive heart disease, or raised blood pressure, the gradient in 1949–1953 was from social class I downwards (123–101). By 1970–1972 it had changed to an upward trend (71–141). No doubt sensitivity to health education and the capacity to attract efficient treatment had contributed to this reversal.

A disturbing fact to emerge is that death rates are tending to level off. For example, between 1951 and 1961 there was a decline in the death rate in social class I. But between 1961 and 1971 this levelled off and there was no further improvement. The principles of healthy living have obviously not permeated our society even in its most perceptive segment and much avoidable disease still prevails.

It is heartening to find in the introduction to the survey the laconic comment – 'Latterly attention has also moved to the psychosocial effects of stress and general occupational conditions –'. This 'attention' seems at present to be rather superficial. For instance there is in the Survey no attempt to compare shift workers with day workers, or workers on a conveyor belt system with self-paced workers, airline pilots with airport ground staff. In other words no comparison is made between work which is inherently stressful with work which is less so. The survey will no doubt become more subtle in time and help to spotlight areas of high occupational stress so that conditions in these areas can be ameliorated. More detailed surveys of the kind mentioned are being carried out by research workers on a small scale as we shall presently see. Meanwhile we can be grateful to the national survey for what it has already achieved.

Occupation and Disease

Let us now turn to the effects of occupation on coronary heart disease. A common finding from several different sources points to the relative immunity of farm workers from this condition as expressed by anginal pain or heart muscle damage. A survey by the Office of Health Economics in 1966[8] reports a far lower consulting rate for these diseases in men aged between fifteen and sixty-four working in agriculture, horticulture and forestry. This applied equally to all levels of work – to the manager, the farmer, and the labourer. The same point is made by Ari Shirom in 1973.[9]

Agricultural workers in a Kibbutz in Israel were compared with white collar workers, craftsmen and factory workers and came off best.

Assembly line work with its forced pacing, its monotony and clamour has often been suspected of responsibility for stress-induced illness, but there is no evidence that it precipitates heart disease. Indeed the contrary has been shown by P. J. Baxter.[10] He examined the frequency of heart attacks in production line and non-production line workers in a factory manufacturing small cars and vans. The fate of some 12,000 men, almost equally divided between the two categories, was reviewed. Significantly more men in the non-production line work were affected, the ratio being 1.54 to 1. One explanation for this rather unexpected finding may be that although assembly line men are under stress the physical work involved protects them from excessive coronary disease. Other investigations have shown that drivers of double-decker buses are more at risk than the clippies on the self-same buses and government clerks are at greater risk than postmen.

There is strong evidence that occupational stress influences coronary heart disease. Henry Russek and Burton Zohman[11] compared a hundred men aged between twenty-five and forty who had had this condition with one hundred healthy controls and found that of the former, no fewer than ninety-one told a story of occupational stress while in the latter group only twenty admitted to that kind of experience. Meyer Friedman and Ray Rosenman[12] reported a peak level of cholesterol in the blood in accountants during their busiest and most harassing month of the year and a corresponding increase in the incidence of coronary heart disease.

L. G. Reeder and his colleagues[13] in a study of Dutch postal services personnel found that the frequency of electrocardiographic abnormalities, pointing in large measure to coronary heart disease, was connected more to the level of responsibility than to the type of work. It did not matter whether the workers were in technical, administrative or postal jobs. What was of importance was the responsibility level of the job. The highest job categories had the greatest ECG changes.

It emerges that coronary heart disease, while being related to occupational stress, is not confined to any particular type of work. It affects workers in all occupations and strikes particularly where responsibility is greatest and the worker feels he is subjected to pressure and harassment. As, however, is apparent from the more cheerful statistics relating to agricultural workers, clippies and physically active postmen, there is the protective value of physical exercise which decreases proneness to coronary heart disease.

When one looks into the effect of occupation on the occurrence of other illness such as high blood pressure and duodenal ulcer a similar picture comes to light. Sidney Cobb and Robert Rose[14] carried out an excellent study on men working in the air transport industry. They compared two groups. The first, air traffic controllers perched in control towers, the second, airmen engaged in actual flight operations. It was thought likely that although both groups were under occupational stress and strain the former would be more continuously on the alert, exposed to even greater responsibilities and suffering more illness in consequence. This assumption proved to be correct. Men in the control towers developed high blood pressure at an earlier age, and four times as frequently as the airmen and, interestingly, those in high density traffic suffered more than those in low density traffic. The same study also looked into the frequency of duodenal ulcer and diabetes in the two groups. As was expected duodenal ulcers were reported twice as frequently in air traffic controllers. The same applied to diabetes but the evidence here was not quite so strong; and again there were more of these illnesses in high traffic density towers where stress levels were undoubtedly greater.

One of us (M.C.) has for some time been interested in the working conditions, stress factors and preventive medicine in air crews and traffic controllers and has carried out several research projects in this area. Investigation of air crews and passengers can be performed by portable, inexpensive and ingenious machines such as the Medilog Recorder (Oxford Instruments) which do not interfere with the subjects' movements and capacity to work. They do not even require the presence of a doctor. The machine measures physiological changes, particularly the electrocardiogram, blood pressure, body temperature, electroencephalogram and other events which can all be synchronized on playback.

The importance of such measurements is that not only can changes in stress hormones be observed but the electroencephalogram can also be recorded to give a true objective measure of fatigue levels. In one experiment on long distance pilots and navigators small sleep patterns, with sleep spindles, were noted at approximately two to three am in aircrew on duty. Urine adrenaline and noradrenaline were raised for up to two to three days after the flight, while plasma cortisol was reduced, suggesting a state of post-flight fatigue. It is presumed that similar conditions occur in air traffic control officers who are not subjected to any time zone changes but only to changes due to shift working. In further work on pilots it was found that it took approximately half the number of days as there are hours in the time zone shift for the body to adapt its hormonal and other rhythms. Thus it takes six to seven days to adapt adequately to a time zone shift of twelve hours. Such considerations are very important in the design of shifts. Dr Melton[15] has reported the instinctive preference of American controllers for a quick two-day changeover system where the body is not given time to change its internal rhythms. It just overrides the change and misses it out. In contrast a continually rotating shift system operates at Heathrow, London, and this is felt to be disruptive and stressful.

Detailed medical evidence, both physiological and biochemical, on the effects of different work schedules is now available and, as already pointed out, there is a high incidence of stress-related disease in air traffic controllers. So it is remarkable that there is such a low level of expenditure on research in the aircraft industry into the functions and maintenance of one of the integral parts of the operating system, the health of the individuals concerned.

The high incidence of disease in air traffic controllers is certainly not due to any inherent defect in their psychological make-up. Karson and O'Dell studied their personality profile and found that in all the essential characteristics it was as sound as, if not sounder than, that of the general population. They were brighter, unusually attentive to detail, they had stronger super egos, they were practical and hard-headed in their approach to life and work and, in particular, they had a low tendency to worry and anxiety.

Among air traffic controllers there appears to be a dislike of work schedule rotation and this is not surprising as it leads to a strain on their powers of adaptation. Moreover some controllers are expected to undertake a task requiring high accuracy and vigilance over a four to five hour period, when even lorry drivers are limited to two hours without a break. While the total hours of duty may not be excessive the way in which they are divided appears to be an important consideration.

It is important in both air traffic controllers and pilots to look for early warning signs of stress-related disorders and to adopt a preventive approach to the maintenance of health. It should be possible to do this without inducing a pathological fear of doctors and medical tests.

Shift Work

One of the horrors of industrial life is the shift system. As automation spreads its tentacles throughout industry, the costly machine must be made to work relentlessly twenty-four hours a day and we, its servants, must be prepared to sacrifice our biological and social habits and tend it round the clock. There is no doubt that the physical and mental health of thousands of shift workers suffers in consequence. Some of the recent findings of research workers in this area are of particular importance to those organizing, and those working in, industry as they will help to formulate a rational approach to shift work (it is after all unavoidable at times), which will assure good use of the machine while fully safeguarding health.

It should be a prime principle of shift work that only those workers who can tolerate it should be asked to undertake it. The work of O. Ostberg[16] is very helpful in this respect. First he makes some very necessary generalizations. Workers suffering from chronic conditions requiring continuous treatment, for example diabetes and epilepsy, are by the nature of their illness unsuitable. Those that require regular meals and especial care with diet, such as peptic ulcer sufferers, should not be asked to do shift work and finally workers with existing heart problems or those already under great stress at home should avoid the additional stress of shift work. He makes a plea for stabilized shift work as opposed to rotating shift work as frequent adaptation from one rhythm to another is harmful. He points out that more night workers will sleep fewer hours than their more fortunate day comrades and that part of the stress of night shifts can be put down to this factor. The research he then describes, concerns some forty-eight men, computer operators and output handlers, who are examined after rotating shiftwork to determine their ease of adaptation to the different shifts. The times of the shifts were 0800, 1600, and 2400 hours and each shift lasted one week. He took into account sleep and wakefulness patterns, round the clock temperature readings, physical fitness and appetite. He also posed a fourteen item questionnaire which divided the workers into those who were comfortable with morning work (showing 'morningness') and those more at ease with evening work (showing 'eveningness'). The best adaptations were judged to have occurred in those whose questionnaires pointed to 'eveningness' working the evening shift and the worst adaptations in those with 'morningness' responses working the night shift. This type of investigation could well open the way to accurate physiological assessment of men's suitability for different kinds of shift work. Those whose time clocks and constitutions would put them at risk should obviously not be asked to work unnatural hours.

The risk factor in shift work is emphasized by the fascinating researches of Töres Theorell and Torbjörn Akerstedt.[17] In Sweden as many as twenty per cent of workers are engaged in shift work and of this group a half are on rotating shifts. In other words ten per cent of workers are particularly at risk, making the problem one of considerable magnitude. The two investigators considered the progress of two groups of railway workers, whose job it was to replace sleepers. Group A consisted of sixteen men who had just completed a night shift (2230-0730 hours) lasting three weeks and were scheduled for three weeks day duty (0730–1630 hours). Group B consisted of seventeen men who were about to do the reverse, ie take on night duty after a spell of day shift. Various chemicals related to stress were measured. Adrenaline and noradrenaline output in twenty-four hours rose to dramatic levels in group B, the one which had taken on the more arduous shift. As for group A, now doing day work, there was no change in the noradrenaline pattern but output of adrenaline fell. This seems to show the challenge of night work and indicates fatigue during the period of recovery from it. Even more striking were the findings of the other indicators of stress and risk. In group B, engaged in night work, blood cholesterol, total fats and sugar rose, while in group A, recovering from night work, these same indices fell. This is not to say that anyone suffered an episode of actual illness but only that these findings suggest an increased risk of developing illness such as coronary heart disease.

We are therefore unwise to play around with shift work to suit the convenience of the machine or the dictates of output or profit.

This type of work may have to be done but with our eyes open to its effects on our biological rhythms and with the adoption of all necessary precautions suggested by the findings of modern research.

As long ago as 1961 Richard C. Browne[18] carried out a profound study on industrial stress and made recommendations which are as valid today as they were then. He found that certain regions, perhaps where living conditions were hardest, for example North-West England and Northern Ireland, had exceptionally high sickness rates; that the older worker suffered from more prolonged bouts of illness; that rheumatism and diseases of the skin ranked second and third in the causes of sickness absence. It was his experience that the greater the size of the department the more illness one could expect. He noticed that night shift workers lost some two hours of sleep daily and that the accident rate was highest at night. Performance fell appreciably between the hours of 7.00 pm and 7.00 am, the first week of night work being especially difficult. He concluded – 'Working at night on a shift system causes more or less biological fatigue, but it may be industrially unavoidable,' and advised 'night work should only be permitted in cases of continuous operation or in war.'

Suggested Policies

After this short review of current thinking on the effects of stress on the health of workers in Industry we return to the problem of how to take practical steps to prevent illness in this field in the light of present day knowledge.

In 1950 the World Health Organization defined occupational health as follows: –

> Occupational health should aim at the promotion and maintenance of the highest degree of physical, mental and social well-being of workers in all occupations; the prevention among workers of departures from health caused by their working conditions; the protection of workers in their employment from risks resulting from factors adverse to health; the placing and maintenance in an occupational environment adapted to his physiological and psychological equipment; and, to summarize; the adaptation of work to man and of each man to his job.

We are a long way from this ideal.

We may be satisfied that where the connection between dangers in the industrial environment and health is straightforward action is constantly being taken. The time has now come to recognize the disturbance to well-being brought about by industrial stress and to tackle the less obvious causes of ill-health in Industry.

Whereas the causes of stress may be social or economic, the effects are mainly medical and this fact justifies the doctor in putting forward suggestions to Industry of a social and economic nature. We have seen that much disease, eg peptic ulcer, mental illness and the Rheumatic disorders is class and income related. It seems that poverty is linked with illness. Therefore it would be logical to give medical support to pressure already being exercised for a minimum wage in Industry. At the other end of the scale it has been shown that a position of privilege in Industry also carries its risks. Men in jobs carrying high responsibility and employers of labour are at risk in respect of coronary heart disease. They too need protection. Perhaps their timetables should be less crowded, they might be encouraged to share or delegate responsibility and they might with profit learn techniques of relaxation.

It should be widely realized that exercise is protective in coronary heart disease. Correction should therefore be made for inactivity in sedentary occupations. Facilities for sports and exercise might be provided in or near the work place with time made available during office hours for their use. Forty minutes per week would be quite sufficient[19] and could easily be borrowed from the working week. It may be argued that almost everyone can make their own arrangements for recreation but sedentary occupation constitutes a work hazard and protection against it should therefore be the employers' responsibility. It may be possible in some occupations which are at present totally sedentary to introduce an element of physical activity, for example by job rotation. And yet again the sedentary worker might be given the opportunity of working in the open for a short part of the year. It may not always make economic sense but it will make health sense.

Rotating shifts have been incriminated for potential ill-health in so many studies that Industry must try to make minimum use of this system. Where it cannot be avoided employees should have a thorough medical check to ascertain their suitability for this type of duty. Far better for a particular worker to maintain his shift hours for some months so that a satisfactory adaptation of the body can be made and the internal clock be adjusted to altered demand.

It has been suggested in the chapters on fatigue that one of the main causes of the rheumatic and allergic complaints is exhaustion. We think it is reasonable at this stage for Industry to take note of this likely relationship between Industrial fatigue and these conditions and to take steps to obviate excessive fatigue in its work force. This should not be too difficult at a time of increasing mechanization, automation and mass unemployment. There should be little resistance on the part of management to the reduction of working hours. Where the job is hard and exacting adequate breaks between work spells could be encouraged. Perhaps the British worker is right to insist on his tea-break. Far better to have a healthy work force putting all their energy and enthusiasm into the task than one which is exhausted and depleted by the inroads of rheumatism and lumbago.

Now that so many women are engaged in Industry we must protect them from the double stress of their family and their work. They already suffer more from rheumatic problems than their husbands. Not only should they be made aware of the dangers of an excessive work load but they should also be helped with shorter hours of work, childminding and other facilities. In this approach we are not 'male chauvinist pigs' but doctors showing rational concern.

We come to the more intangible problem of mental stress at work. Alexis Brook[20] has divided this into three stages. The first, an early, preventable state for which responsibility lies at the door of management. The second stage is more advanced. Morale may have dropped and some individuals may have developed minor symptoms. In the third stage there are clear cut symptoms of physical, mental and behavioural disorders. It is too late for preventive action on the part of management. Brook considers that 'increasing attention is now being given to what is called the social responsibility of business and industry.'

A lot of thought has gone into job design[21] to satisfy both the requirements of Industry and the social and personal requirements of the worker. By giving careful attention to the needs of the individual worker many potential emotional troubles can be prevented.

To avoid boredom and fatigue there should be sufficient variety within the job. Yet too much variety may lead to insufficient skill in the task and consequent inefficiency and frustration.

If possible the worker should feel that he is making a worthwhile contribution to the final product and that his skill and effort are appreciated by the industry and by the community.

There should be outlets for the expression of grievances and for communication of ideas which contribute to work efficiency and work satisfaction. The worker should be involved in the setting of standards of quantity and quality and should know what progress is being made by adequate feedback.

In the nature of things there will be conflict and competition between groups and among groups in Industry. This is both inevitable and necessary. But much avoidable stress in Industry is brought about by poor labour relations. The conflict between management and labour simmers on through a long tradition of confrontation and boils over from time to time causing chronic states of resentment, anxiety and anger and undoubtedly contributing to ill-health. Some social and political steps need to be taken to remove the sources of conflict and tension between the various sectors of industry. Whether it be by worker participation in management, by profit sharing, by worker co-operatives, by improved communication between management and labour, by whatever means, industrial peace and reduced tension must be brought about. These measures, if successful, will probably bring about great economic benefits but the improvement in health will be even greater.

13

The Birth of Anxiety

AS WITH ALL HUMAN EMOTIONS, anxiety has a positive as well as a negative value whether looked at from the point of view of performance, motivation or survival, and God forbid that we should wish to tamper with it except when it becomes pathological, when it no longer contributes to survival but leads to illness and self-destruction. An understanding, if this were possible, of the genesis of anxiety, of its serviceable limits and of the ways it could be curbed when out of hand would be useful tools for almost everyone in society from laymen to doctors.

One of the assets of anxiety is said to be its ability to improve performance. The public speaker, the musician, the athlete awaiting his event all suffer from it and all declare that without it they would not give their best. The theory runs as follows. In the absence of anxiety there will be no tension, no alertness and an uninspired performance; with adequate anxiety performance will be at peak level, while with excess anxiety there will be too widespread a response including contradictory and futile activities, inevitably leading to a decline in performance. We are only partly in agreement with this concept which is surely based on too broad a definition of anxiety. There is need to separate anxiety from states of tension and excitement. *The Encyclopedia of Psychiatry for General Practitioners*[1] defines anxiety as 'An unpleasant emotional experience, varying in degree from mild unease to intense dread, associated with the anticipation of impending or future disaster.' This is an excellent description of true anxiety and puts the accent on the element of possible failure or disaster. When facing a test, whether physical or mental, we are naturally aroused, alert and excited. In many instances there will, in addition, be the fear of failure and consequent anxiety but this is surely not universal. So we would like to see physiological preparedness and excitement separated from anxiety. In other words anxiety need not be a necessary condition for a good performance.

The other positive values of anxiety are fairly self-evident. Without an element of fear and foreboding we would rush blindly into dangerous situations. Anxiety acts as a brake to precipitate action, causes us to reflect and to take carefully chosen and appropriate action. Children are subject to parental and school guidance and correction when they engage in unsocial acts. Later this external control is interiorized and the growing child learns to have its own standards of right and wrong, some modelled on the behaviour of adults, others in reaction to their example. So an anxiety is generated to try to live up to these standards and this is a socially useful emotion which encourages social conformity without external sanctions. On the other hand the amoral child may have fear of punishment but it will, regrettably, have no anxiety about social wrong doing.

There are many different explanations and interpretations of anxiety and we would like to quote some of these from Arthur Jersild's book on Child Psychology.[2] According to Soren Kirkegaard, anxiety is related to concepts of self. If there is self-fulfilment, although the fulfilment is poor and limited there will be satisfaction and, presumably, no anxiety. He wrote in 1949 – 'Even what one might call the poorest personality is everything when he has chosen himself, for the great thing, is not to be this or that but to be oneself.' It is the frustration of not being allowed to be oneself which leads to inner conflict and anxiety. One might comment on this view that the anxiety for self-fulfilment is attractive and even laudable providing it does not prevent the self-fulfilment of others.

A rather similar approach is made by Hoskey. The passage is written so eloquently that it deserves restating.

> A chronic condition of anxiety develops when a child has to build defences against an environment that is unreliable, unjust and harsh, an environment that he does not have power to change, which undermines his ability to place trust in himself. He is not simply frightened in this or that particular of his life, but the environment as a whole is a menace, threatening his individuality, and interfering with his opportunity to develop his potentialities as a person. Such a forbidding environment exists when a child is unloved and is treated without consideration.

Few of us are able to follow the complexities of the analytic approach to anxiety. However it has pervaded our thinking and some mention must be made of it. Sigmund Freud apparently differentiated between separation anxiety in which a dependent child finds himself unable to cope in the absence of his mother, and the anxiety of inner conflict between the need for gratification of one's instincts and conditions which forbid this. Jersild quotes a rather involved example of Freud's: the case of Hans and his phobia of horses. Hans apparently suffered from an unresolved Oedipus complex. He felt a desire to displace his father and possess his mother. This was a feeling he must naturally repress. The forbidden thought induced in him a fear of his father whom he also loved. Apparently his hostility and fear towards his father were rerouted to the same emotions towards horses. It is not easy to explain the transfer from father to horse but apparently he had seen a horse injured. We might end by agreeing with the principles which Freud expresses without necessarily accepting this particular case history which seems to contain both common sense and fantasy.

Fear is both a precursor of anxiety and one of its ingredients. It is said to relate to an actual and tangible threat whereas anxiety is less specific, more nebulous and relates to presumed or future threats. Fear is a more conscious mental state, an acknowledged dread, while anxiety lies more often in the subconscious and its cause may be hidden from the sufferer. If we are going to look for the causes of anxiety it might be useful to explore first the causes of fear as this is the simpler and more straightforward emotion.

There are primary fears which do not need to be learnt, such as fears of loud noises, of pain or injury, of sudden loss of physical support or balance, of disagreeable or irritating smells, of separation from a parent and so on. These are the earliest fears of the infant. But even they are not absolute. The threshold of what constitutes a disturbance, and brings on fear, varies from infant to infant. A stimulus, such as a loud noise may be unbearable to one infant but is well tolerated by the other. There is then, even at this early stage, an inborn difference of response. The thresholds for arousal and fear are not identical. Then grafted onto these come acquired or learnt fears – fears by association, such as fear of insects which sting, dogs which bite, flames which burn. Added to this are the fears of scolding and punishment for disapproved forms of behaviour. The list grows and the precipitating factors become more complex. There follow fear of being ridiculed, of loss of status and self-esteem, of work security and so on indefinitely.

What factors then are going to increase the likelihood of acquiring fear and what factors in reducing it or limiting it to reasonable bounds, what in any case is 'reasonable' in this context. Where a fear is based on a real threat and is a protective mechanism then surely it is reasonable. Where it is based on imaginary or exaggerated threats it is unreasonable and might then be placed into the category of pathological fear or anxiety.

The child that is unlikely to suffer from an excess of fear is one who has a secure home, secure parental affection, and rational, stable, dependable guidance. There will be within this broad generalization, children, who by reason of real handicaps, either mental or physical, will have more cause for fear and who will be frightened in spite of adequate and reassuring parental behaviour. Disparagement saps confidence and the child which is constantly criticized and never praised, reacts with timidity, fear and anxiety. Illness may bring on fear by weakening a child, but also because he may regard the incident as due to his own fault or carelessness. He had after all been told not to get wet or cold or come into contact with certain forbidden things. So may come an element of guilt which adds to fear.

There are enough genuine threats to security in the world without the creation of imaginary or false threats. Since speech began, parents have attempted to encourage a dread and foreboding of the supernatural and mythical either unwittingly or expressedly to intimidate their children into obedience. Human beings have invented hell, devils, sorcerers and witches, gremlins, ghosts, robots and now even monsters from outer space to 'instil' fear into themselves and their children. In societies where these beliefs are widely held neurotic fear is rampant. It would be invidious to point a finger at any particular race for, in this respect, the developed nations vie with the undeveloped. In some countries these primitive customs and beliefs are cloaked in deceptively civilized processes, and rationalized by a philosophical veneer; but the underlying myth can easily be exposed. It is desperately necessary to limit fear to the real threats which surround us so abundantly and discard our primitive creations of hell, sin and chastisement by all manner of imaginary objects. Our children will sleep more peacefully in bed and their dreams will be less nightmarish.

As Jersild points out, it is no joke when a child is told about hell, and is led to believe that he may land up there unless he behaves. How can he distinguish between fact and fantasy? In this hell he will not only be desperately uncomfortable, but will, in addition be separated from his parents – a possibility he cannot face. So what right has anyone to inflict this horrible fantasy on a child?

Fear and anxiety are in many cases due to an information gap. One need hardly elaborate. A traveller in a strange land will not be afraid provided he has had previous information that there are no hostile bands and that food, water and shelter will be freely available. A patient awaiting an operation will be calmer if the details of the procedure have been fully explained.

Vicarious exposure through the media, which are becoming ever more immediate and realistic, to violence, danger and catastrophe, opens up new possibilities for fear.

Fear seems to stalk in certain families. Children of fearful parents acquire their own fear through two channels. On the one hand they may inherit a sensitive and vulnerable brain mechanism and endocrine system and on the other they will learn a faulty behaviour pattern by example and imitation. As with the argument on the relative role of heredity and environment in intelligence so there is the same dispute over the part played by these factors in anxiety. It would be pleasant to think that a large part of anxiety is acquired and that, in consequence, it would be amenable to correction but we know too little to be dogmatic on this subject. Even if hereditary factors were responsible for anxiety to the tune of sixty to eighty per cent, as is suspected in the case of intelligence, environmental factors are sufficiently obtrusive for there to be ample room for efforts at their correction.

Turning to another perspective on the study of acquired anxiety we can derive some help from experimental and anecdotal evidence. A most striking example of acquired fear was the famous case of Pavlov's dogs. His experimental animals who had had considerable training in various conditioning procedures, were, one day, suddenly exposed to a violent storm and flood in which they were almost drowned. By good fortune they were rescued from death in the nick of time, but only after some had reached a state of collapse. It was noticed after the ordeal that those who had collapsed, but not the others, had lost all their recent conditioning and had acquired a chronic state of fear and terror of the sound of running water. The two elements of this new conditioning were first, the intensity of the experience and second, the state of collapse.

The anxiety neurosis of shell-shocked soldiers develops under similar conditions of intense fear and collapse.

A useful experimental model of anxiety is the Conditional Emotional Response (CER). Neal Miller[3] reported his work on the 'Psychosomatic effects of specific types of training' in 1969. In it, he made use of variations in the CER to demonstrate variations in the degree of generalized fear provoked and variations in the secondary psychosomatic symptoms and lesions. Small, measured electric shocks were applied to the tails of rats, this was the unconditioned stimulus. The warning, conditioned stimulus used was a light. Four groups of rats were trained in different ways. The first group was warned of the impending shock by a bright light. The second by a weak light. In other words the shock was predictable in both groups but more plainly in the former. The third group was exposed to both lights and shocks but in a totally irregular and unpredictable manner, while the fourth group received only shocks but no light signal at all. No drink was allowed during the shock training but water was provided during the test trial which followed. Fear would inhibit the rats from drinking and the degree of their fear could be measured by the quantitative reduction in the amount drunk. As might be expected the group, well warned by a strong light, suffered least fear and drank most. A weak warning was less successful in reducing fear while unpredictable shocks brought about the greatest degree of fear. This work beautifully supports the psychological premise that unpredictability or an information gap are potent factors in the genesis of fear.

Further work in Miller's laboratory resulted in similar findings in relation to avoidability and coping. It had been noticed that pilots of combat aircrafts developed less fear and less illness than co-pilots and this had led to speculation that the ability to take avoiding action was useful in regulating and decreasing fear. The co-pilots were exposed to the same dangers as pilots but, not being in control, they would feel helpless and react with anxiety. In the experiment rats were paired and were given signalled tail shocks. One member of the pair could turn off the shock either after its onset or, by turning off the signal, he could even avoid shock altogether. The other rat could do nothing to avert the shock but had to rely on his companion. A third rat was let off lightly and subjected only to the warning signal but no shock. Rats that could avoid shock started to drink earlier than their helpless partners. Here then was experimental confirmation that the option of an avoidance response reduces generalized fear.

Miller and his colleagues did not stop at this but went on to show that greater fear led to more extensive psychosomatic symptoms and organ strain or damage. For example rectal temperature can be taken as a measure of increased stress and metabolic turnover. The rectal temperature in control rats given no shock at all remained unaltered. In those that received a signalled shock it rose only to a moderate extent, 1.7° centigrade, while in rats exposed to greater stress, that of unsignalled shocks, there was the greatest rise, 2.1° centigrade. By similar experiments they demonstrated that in this species greater fear was associated with larger stomach ulcers and greater weight loss.

Animals can be taught behavioural patterns through fear or they can be conditioned by reward. Whereas fear inhibits activity, pleasure strengthens it. In suitably rewarded dogs the immediately preceding activity can be strengthened. In this way they can be made to salivate more copiously, to increase or decrease their heart rate, to contract or relax their intestine. In one experiment on a rat Miller, to his great delight, succeeded in bringing about contraction of blood vessels in one ear and dilatation of these vessels in the other. Nowadays one would not be surprised if the exponents of Yoga could do the same.

Some other factors are known to influence the acquisition of anxiety. Gay Gaer Luce, in her fascinating book *Body Time*,[4] discusses the work of Charles F. Stroebel on the effect of the circadian rhythm on the learning of fear. He has shown in rats that fear is acquired more quickly when the blood cortisol levels are at their peak, in the early part of the night or dark period when they are most active. He was able to demonstrate a similar effect in monkeys who have a circadian cortisol rhythm akin to man's with high early morning levels. So it is likely that fear will enter a human being's mind more readily in the early morning or at times of stress when his blood cortisol is raised and such a hypothesis may help to explain the soldier's acquired anxiety at the height of battle. In the *Anatomy of Fear* Lord Moran describes many an occasion when a previously intrepid soldier, shelled ferociously at the height of battle excitement, succumbs to a fear which remains engraved upon him.

When Stroebel flattened out the cortisol curve by the use of metyrapone, a substance which interferes with the synthesis of cortisol, he induced a uniform rate of acquiring fear throughout the twenty-four hours.

Another way of looking at the problem of fear is to consider the manner in which it can be extinguished or lost. An individual may possess an unusual parcel of fear either by acquiring it too readily or by losing it too sparingly. Excessive anxiety is counter-productive as it leads to excessive expenditure of energy. In Duffy's view[5] all behaviour has a common dimension of energy release. The response to any given situation is proportional to the degree of effort the organism considers necessary. A permanent state of high arousal and anxiety will lead to an excessive response and will be wasteful or even harmful. In order to avoid unnecessary activity and save energy animals have, in the course of evolution, developed the physiological mechanism of habituation. This ensures that the response to a non-threatening stimulus is extinguished. It would indeed be a bore, and harmful at that, if the investigatory response of animals, described by Pavlov over fifty years ago and, now grandly named the 'orienting reaction' were repeated endlessly in response to a repetitive but harmless signal. Malcolm H. Lader,[6] has carried out a considerable amount of research on this subject and has greatly increased our appreciation of its significance in mental illness and psychosomatic disease.

The orienting reaction is the basis of an animal's response to changes in the environment. This reaction comprises a series of activities. First there are changes in the end organs which analyse the environment, then changes in the muscles controlling the sense organs to allow them to follow movements in the environment. Attention is thus riveted onto the disturbing stimulus. When its nature has been interpreted and evaluated there follow changes in muscle tone and posture in keeping with the intended response, changes in brain activity and finally autonomic adjustments.

It is by studying these adjustments that research workers can assess the degree of habituation which takes place. Disturbing stimuli are accompanied by an increase in pulse rate, rise in blood pressure, an increased galvanic skin response (GSR), increased forearm blood flow (FBF), electroencephalographic changes and so on. The GSR and FBF need some explanation. When the skin is dry, electrical conductivity is poor, but in anxiety the skin becomes moist and, as the resistance drops, so conductivity increases. This test can be used as a lie detector. The liar, disturbed by his sense of guilt and fear, sweats more profusely and gives himself away. In a similar fashion anxiety (by stimulating sympathetic cholinergic vasodilator fibres) increases the forearm blood flow which can be measured by a special plethysmograph or strain gauge.

Lader found that habituation was linked to the state of arousal. A high level of arousal would result – as is to be expected – in slow habituation, while a low level was related to rapid habituation. In keeping with this drugs with a tranquillizing effect such as Equanil and Largactil, accelerated habituation. Drugs possessing a stimulant effect, like amphetamine, delayed habituation. It would appear then that measures to lower the arousal level such as the use of tranquillizers or perhaps simple relaxation techniques will lead to a more rapid reduction of the level of fear and anxiety.

Extroverts, by definition, focus their attention more on the outside world and less on their subjective feelings while the reverse is the case in introverts and this may account for the increased sensitivity of the latter and lead perhaps to a lower threshold of arousal. Whatever the mechanism, Lader found that introverts habituate less rapidly than extroverts.

When we look at anxiety we find that those who suffer from this common and distressing symptom habituate slowly or not at all. So there is a relationship between anxiety and habituation; but which should be regarded as the cart, and which the horse? Lader puts it that anxiety retards habituation, but one could equally well say that poor habituation leads to anxiety. In other words if one cannot lose a conditioned fear one remains anxious.

Anxiety can be very localized, as in patients who suffer from an isolated phobia to, say, birds or spiders; or it might be more widespread as is the case with some social phobias, or agoraphobia, where the patient has a fear of going outside the home into, as it appears to him or her, the terrifying outer world, or again the anxiety might be free floating and attach itself to all or any activity. Well now, habituation takes place normally in the first category, that of the isolated phobia, and is slowed down in the case of the more widespread phobias.

In the psychosocial field, the ability to acclimatize to a horrifying experience can be tested by the use of films. A mixed audience was shown the same films with a violent and frightening content on two occasions at an interval of one week. Lader demonstrated that those with a low anxiety rating habituated well as far as autonomic activity was concerned, while those with a high anxiety rating did not habituate and even showed some increase in autonomic activity. He concludes that habituation, the ability not to respond in a stereotyped manner to repetitive stimuli, is a valuable asset, and this advantage is lost in states of high arousal and raised anxiety. Such a loss is not only wasteful of energy and a bar to efficiency, it can also be harmful to health by reason of excessive activity of the autonomic nervous system.

If the speed of habituation is relevant to anxiety, can we do anything to bring about an acceleration? This seems, at first sight, to be a tall order, but it is not as far-fetched as it might appear. The state of arousal can be lowered, with a partial shift towards the desired effect, by the use of calming drugs and relaxation, and modern behaviour therapy, while making use of these measures, goes further and achieves habituation to an ascending hierarchy of phobic states. This form of therapy is now beginning to be so well known to the public that it needs only a very brief comment. The phobia is analysed and its components are arranged in order of severity. The least frightening element is dealt with first and the more troublesome are then tackled in sequence. Habituation is achieved by linking the feared object to a pleasant and reassuring atmosphere, ie making a rewarding rather than a frightening association. This being a harmless and relatively successful form of therapy it is a thousand pities that it is not more readily available.

We have talked at some length about the birth of anxiety as if it were the only emotion worthy of study. This is far from the case. Although anxiety may be the most harmful emotion there are many runners up such as anger, guilt and jealousy. The enormous range of emotions has not been discussed for several reasons. Firstly, most emotions are not clear cut single entities but are composites. If one takes the analogy of colour one can obtain the extraordinary range of subtle colour which is to be found in nature and art by mixing the correct blend of the bold, somewhat coarse, primary colours. In the same way emotions are a blend of primary emotions and we need therefore not discuss the whole range but only the more outstanding primitive ones.

If then we take the emotions associated with escape we are dealing with fear, anxiety, terror, guilt, horror, disgust and so on. But each of these has a component of fear and so only fear and its slightly more complex sister, anxiety, need to be discussed. When emotions involved in attack, such as hate, resentment, disapproval and jealousy, are analysed we find there is a component of anger in all these states and anger alone need be considered. This approach is also legitimate for emotions related to disengagement like boredom, apathy and disinterest. In this scheme of things depression is difficult to place. It has in it elements of self-criticism, lack of self-esteem, worthlessness, sense of failure, anger inwardly directed, anxiety, lack of pleasure, apathy, lack of motivation and fatigue. It is a highly complex mix in which the main ingredients may be anxiety, depletion of brain cell energy and intellectual demoralization. It must be put into a category of its own.

Then there are all the pleasurable emotions, which are likewise combinations, in different proportions, of the primitive emotions of approval but, although modern work tends to show that they may play a small part in psychosomatic disease, we are not going to regard them as particularly traumatic and so can neglect them.

The emotions described are of a personal nature, felt entirely as individuals, but we also appear to exhibit group emotions. So there could be said to be group loyalty, courage, aggression, obedience, panic and so on. These too need not be discussed in detail as they are probably elaborations of personal emotion, with an added touch of hysteria or hypnotic suggestion.

Secondly, we must admit that anxiety in animals is fairly easy to observe and study. It is expressed in the form of retreat, the discontinuance of normal activity and various physiological responses, including a rise in pulse rate and adrenaline production. Anger is more difficult to study. It may be that fear and anger sometimes coexist and we are only aware of the predominant emotion. Many experimental workers talk of the conditioned emotional response, which embraces elements both of fear and anger, rather than the conditioned anxiety response.

Finally we might excuse ourselves for not writing about anger by claiming that the principles which apply to anxiety may apply in large measure to anger as well. Perhaps anger is bred in a similar manner to anxiety in conditions of lack of security, of love and of stable guidance; and habituation to unpleasant stimuli can be encouraged in the angry as it can in the anxious.

14

Bringing Anxiety to Heel

ARE WE IN A POSITION to use the knowledge that there is in this relatively poorly charted field of the emotions in order to reduce some of the personal burden of anxiety, guilt, aggression and the wide range of other harmful emotions which are thought to lead to so much mental and physical misery and ill-health? This is still a debatable proposition. Charles A. Roberts in his paper on the Primary Prevention of Psychiatric Disorders[1] considers that the effort should be made, and would be successful. He writes – 'If we ever devote the same concentration of energy and resources to people as we have to our physical environment we will find a solution.' The trend of progressive thinking supports him. We have come to realize that we have worshipped technology and the machine more than they deserve and now, for various reasons, including our increasing awareness of the hardships which the Industrial Revolution has imposed upon the workers and our appreciation that material things are dominating us, many people are converted to the notion that interpersonal relationships and personal mental contentedness are more important than the acquisition of wealth. The time is therefore ripe for a greater understanding of mental processes and an attempt at the control of faulty emotional attitudes and responses.

Intervention is possible at many different levels and through many different agencies. Basically mental health will depend on motivation and understanding. Motivation there is to a considerable degree. Many people are searching for ways and means of achieving inner peace. In the past it has been possible to attain this in religious belief and practice, in stable families and communities, in the observance of long standing social customs and traditions. But as many of the traditional means of seeking peace and security have been eroded or found wanting under present conditions there is a renewed search for answers to this everlasting problem. Perhaps the answer does not lie in a system imposed upon us, in accepting the teachings of this or that philosopher or sage but in greater faith in ourselves, coupled with a greater understanding of the wonderful biological structures that are within us. Then will follow the full use of our individual potential, the best functioning of our brains and bodies and a respect both for ourselves and for all our fellow creatures. A respect based on the appreciation of what we and others can achieve. In short, many of our gods have failed us and it may be that we are now prepared to examine ourselves to see what strengths are within us.

If this is so then there will come about a demand for information. The media are not backward in this respect. Both in sound and vision there is a flow of material on the brain, on body structure and function, and on interpersonal relationships. Writers are making a steady contribution as evidenced by the work of Erwin Lausch, Arthur Koestler, Alvin Toffler, Hans Eysenck and many others. The medical profession perhaps lags behind in some ways as it tries to cope with vast reservoirs of personal unhappiness and maladjustment on a one to one basis. Admittedly Group therapy is a means of enlarging the range of therapeutic effect but even so it is not preventive in the true sense as patients are admitted to treatment after they have already broken down. Should doctors not take part on a larger scale in health education? What efforts are being made to enlarge the activities of the Health Education Council in the field of mental health? Could not doctors hold group meetings with their patients on mental health, psychological problems, interpersonal relationships before they break down? Could they not attempt to introduce some of these topics into schools?

Teachers are well aware that some of their pupils are losing interest in conventional education and that apathy and truancy are increasing. Could not the curriculum be made more relevant to their actual lives and to contain practical subjects and ideals which have meaning to them? Amongst other things should not the direction of educational effort be more towards the understanding of our biological selves and healthy social interrelationships? Should our youngsters not be taught more about conflict and harmony in marriage, parenthood and in wider social relationships? Could we not obtain greater maturity in our school leavers through greater understanding of human emotions and greater insight into behaviour and motivation?

Intervention in emotional development is probably of greatest value in infancy and childhood. W. W. Lewis is quoted in C. A. Robert's paper –

> The treatment procedures used in child guidance clinics are based implicitly on two hypotheses – the continuity Hypothesis, that emotional disturbance in a child is symptomatic of a continuing psychological process that may lead to an adult mental illness – the Intervention Hypothesis, therapeutic intervention enhances the child's present adjustment and reduces the likelihood that he will experience serious mental problems in later life.

Although this statement refers to Child Guidance Clinics it is of course applicable to all children with emotional problems. Moreover one may add that by correcting emotional problems at an early stage one not only influences mental health but physical health as well for the two cannot be separated.

From what has been said in the chapter on the emotions certain basic attitudes and approaches emerge towards the development of a sound personality free from excessive anxiety. One of the basic points to appreciate is that emotional malfunctioning need not be fatalistically accepted but, as with all mental processes, is amenable to outside influence and correction. Animal experiment has demonstrated again and again that emotional responses, both of fear linked with avoidance and of pleasure with approval and trust, can be inculcated. Another basic statement would be that fear, anxiety, aggression and the rest of the spectrum have their positive value and no attempt should or can be made to eradicate them. Only where there is excess or distortion should intervention be considered.

The concept of self-fulfilment at different levels is a useful one. As long as a child develops its own potential and is praised for the talents and attitudes it possesses, while having a realistic goal of the possibilities of its own personal attainments, it will be happy and will not suffer guilt or jealousy.

If it is accepted that parental love, security, stable guidance, predictable behaviour and encouragement are vital factors in sound emotional development without undue anxiety then it follows that where parents do not possess the attributes which permit them to give their children this environment then society should, without blaming or moralizing, help to make good this deficiency at the earliest possible moment. These children may, for example, be sent to special nurseries or schools where the teacher-pupil ratio is high and the staff are equipped to deal with emotional problems. Perhaps there should be a monitoring of emotional development in children; it is certainly possible to confront infants with situations which will test their emotional responses or discover by play or questioning whether there is an unnatural quotient of fear and anxiety. Where the emotional balance is patently wrong, where the content of fear, anxiety, aggression or apathy is too great, remedial steps should be taken. We will not attempt to go into the methods to be used which fall into the province of child psychiatrists and child guidance clinics. Our main point is that we should not wait for breakdown but should assess development at different milestones in a child's life and be prepared to take effective and, if necessary, expensive steps to correct abnormalities.

Then society as a whole can take various measures to encourage healthy emotional development. In our view we should erase from our day-to-day lives false and terrifying mythologies. There will, admittedly, be some loss of poetic and literary material. We may feel we are being robbed of a heritage of culture. This is not, however, to suggest a bonfire upon which the offending literary material should be burnt, but only a lessening of emphasis on the occult, a relegation of witchcraft, of devils and hell and suchlike to literary curiosities and not to their use as the bread and butter upon which children are fed. There is also need to lessen the vicarious horror and aggression of which our media are so fond. They will, of course, have to present other forms of excitement and adventure to fill the gaps which are left. We should not be afraid of taking the initiative and insisting that our commercially motivated purveyors of violence, of senseless Frankenstein science fiction remove their hideous rubbish from the screen and replace these things with stories that are more intelligent, more truthful and more in keeping with our potential humanity. There is, of course, argument about the harm which vicarious violence does but it would seem obvious that we are unlikely to adopt a behaviour pattern which we have never seen or experienced, while we have a tremendous propensity to imitation and are likely to make use of patterns of violence which have been presented to us. Freedom of expression need not go so far as to produce generations of anxiety and guilt laden human beings prone to useless violence. No one would object to documentary or other films which tell the truth and depict man with all his faults but, for heaven's sake, let us not invent additional violence and crimes.

Ignorance may lead to fear. It cannot, unfortunately, be claimed that knowledge always eradicates fear, it will only lessen it and reduce it to realistic proportions. It is therefore our duty, in our endeavour to reduce fear in people's lives, to educate children to their full potential and give each other all the information we can in our daily transactions.

The industrial scene is the arena in which perpetual conflicts are fought out between management and worker and between rival elements in both groups. If there should be a need for understanding of conflict and the emotions which are aroused in its wake, it is in this sphere and we should all be content that the subject of Industrial Relations is at last getting the attention it deserves. We are probably going to be less satisfied with the pace of this study and the applications of the principles which emerge from it. It is in this field that so much anxiety, leading to mental and physical disease, is generated and the problem should be tackled at this point and not, after illness has become established, in hospital or in the doctor's surgery.

There are certain situations which should alert us to the possible onset of anxiety, and certain personalities, which by common consent, are more vulnerable to breakdown. Where life change has been too rapid or too catastrophic we may expect emotional derailment and psychosomatic illness. Where there is a state of helplessness, and the individual cannot escape from terror or defend himself adequately, as in conditions of Civil War, the same outcome can be expected. The introspective individual, as was shown by Lader, is less able to habituate and more prone to anxiety. It is in cases of this sort that society should be more ready to intervene to prevent emotional breakdown.

Society has accepted war as inevitable. In so doing it has accepted the physical and mental mutilations which result from it, and all around we find men and women bearing the mental scars of their experience, predominantly those of chronic fear and anxiety. Clinical examples abound and include disordered action of the heart, phobias of all kinds, hypochondriacs, damaged, ineffective personalities and numerous psychosomatic illnesses which lead as often as not to chronic invalidism and unemployment. Add to the war veterans, the victims of concentration camps and civil disturbances and we see a picture of human wreckage strewn about the world. If we are sincere in our desire to decrease fear and anxiety then we should be equally concerned in studying the causes of conflict and war and eliminating this extraordinary behaviour, which we do not share with the bulk of the animal world, from our range of the acceptable. Even though we are surrounded by horrifying conflict, a glimmer of hope can be seen in the efforts of some politicians, university departments and medical groups which are now devoting their energies to the study of war and peace.

Apart from the general measures which we have been considering are there specialized procedures of value in prevention or cure of anxiety? Well of course there are many, some more successful than others and all depending for their success on the skill with which they are applied. Regretfully, one cannot at this moment, be impressed by the quality or quantity of recovery from the anxiety-states and phobias. Admittedly there are mild cases which recover either with the passage of time or with short periods of relatively superficial treatment. But the really severe, chronic anxiety states and phobias seem resistant to the most intense efforts and turn up like bad pennies in doctors' surgeries as a reminder of their lack of effective treatment. We believe the future holds out far greater hope.

A brief case history of a patient suffering from a chronic anxiety state will illustrate both the origin of his illness and its obstinate resistance to treatment.

'A', a thick-set Spaniard of sixty-six, had been through the horrors of the Spanish Civil War. Despite this experience he joined the Allied forces and suffered more combat stress. His personality and health did not break down till he developed a perforated duodenal ulcer while serving as a kitchen hand, in this country. Then he entered a phase of severe anxiety, depression and hypochondriasis associated with physical disabilities such as a high blood pressure, rapid pulse and various rheumatic complaints. These symptoms persisted in spite of efforts by psychiatrists, general practitioners and specialists of all kinds till he finally died many years later of a cancer.

The emotional trauma through which soldiers pass is not appreciated by everyone and their psychiatric difficulties do not get the attention they deserve. Those that break down in combat are obviously removed from the front line and often treated successfully, but lesser degrees of breakdown, which the soldier does his best to hide, are not sought out and it is considered natural that thousands of men leave the forces with some degree of anxiety which, of course, they may keep for the rest of their lives. Then later, as some future stress situation develops, the more recently acquired anxiety joins with the suppressed anxiety to produce serious disability. The General Practitioner will recognize numerous cases of cumulative anxiety in his war veterans. This hidden anxiety in ex-soldiers should, in our opinion, be treated at an early stage. In stressed soldiers a period of convalescence after war service might be useful. During this time they would be encouraged to retell their traumatic experiences either in Group discussion or abreaction. Tranquillizers of a non-addictive nature could be given for short periods and they could perhaps be taught relaxation techniques. If there were an element of disordered action of the heart because of sympathetic overdrive the β Blockers could be used.

It is of course society's duty to think carefully before committing its young men to war, but, having decided on war, it is then its duty to rehabilitate its soldiers not only physically which it does as best it can, but also mentally, which it has so far failed to do.

In the face of such a case how can one have the effrontery to talk of specific measures to lessen anxiety and its companion emotions. Well, it seems to be a case of recognizing anxiety before it gains a permanent foothold and treating it before it has affected personality functions on a wide front and in chronic form. There is usually a crisis point which should be appreciated of the type already described, such as a frightening experience in war or civil conflict, an accident, interpersonal conflict or whatever. It is at this stage that proper measures should be taken, sparing no effort – heavy sedation, adequate rest and rehabilitation. During the last war William Sargant[2] was highly successful with abreaction. The patient would be given an intravenous injection of a barbiturate or of amphetamine and encouraged to relive his horrible experiences. He would reach a point of high excitement, which it was hoped would be followed by collapse. At this point the patient would enter a type of trance state in which he was highly amenable to suggestion. The traumatic memory would lose its power over him and he could be cured. This form of treatment must, of course, remain in the hands of experts but, as it is undoubtedly useful, it should be more widely applied. Sargant found that it was not necessary to recall the actual hurtful experience. Abreaction of imaginary events, allowing the release of strong emotions was likewise beneficial. It appears that the state of trance and increased suggestibility can also be brought about by long continued, repetitive stimuli as in tribal ritual dance and song followed eventually by collapse. Sargant tells the story of an African tribe which, as it was constantly threatened, had to remain on a war footing and high state of preparedness. The young men were indoctrinated to believe that they must all be warriors and forgo the pleasures of marriage and family. Only the older men were permitted wives. This, being an unnatural state, was highly resented. However a dramatic means of enforcing the tribal custom was at hand. At regular intervals there would be tribal gatherings at which with monotonous, exhausting dance and song, the legend was endlessly repeated and the young exhorted to do their duty. The majority succumbed to the hypnotic suggestion. The recalcitrant few were invited to leave the village and were never seen again.

Abreaction is not universally successful. It bestows no lasting relief if the personality of the patient has always been neurotic and unstable even before the stressful event. If the patient is afflicted by a deep depression it is not possible to release anger and fear and so no improvement can be brought about. In these cases it is essential to deal first with the depression. Where an abreaction results in laughter, as the predominant emotion, it fails. Laughter may prevent breakdown but will not relieve it.

Is there any scientific explanation of abreaction? A partial understanding, in general terms, exists but it does not as yet go into details of neuronal function in biochemical and electrical terms. Pavlov described four types of dogs: strong excitatory, showing excessive excitement to minor upsetting stimuli; controlled excitatory, reacting with controlled excitement or aggression; stable plethoric, remaining stable, under all sorts of stressful situations and finally weak inhibitory, reacting with a short period of excitement followed by progressive and finally paralysing inhibition of normal brain function, that is – a protective inhibition. Pavlov held the view that if an animal's nervous system was stimulated transmarginally, beyond its capacity to respond normally, then inhibition sets in, breakdown occurring sooner in the two more vulnerable types, the strong excitatory and weak inhibitory. In the incident where his dogs were nearly drowned and collapsed after a period of great fear and stress, the collapse represented, in part, this stage of inhibition. Similarly in the more recent situation of abreaction this may end in collapse signifying the same reaction. The brain abdicates and a new emotional setting is brought about by suggestion. Repressed and highly traumatic memories are allowed to come back into the normal stream of consciousness. Sargant describes the abreaction as 'Psychologically induced shock treatment.' He considers that the trance state can be produced in two ways, by bringing about 'sensorial excitement' either using strong and abrupt stimuli or fainter and long continued ones. According to him hypnotic suggestion is an allied mechanism. The hypnotic state can be induced by abrupt stimuli as was Charcot's* practice (he would use a bright light or intense noise after subjecting the patient to a period of time in a dark room), or by gentler long continued stimuli.

It would seem to us that fear can be acquired through mechanisms similar to the hypnotic state and can be dispelled using the same techniques.

Sargant writes:

> Excitement and stresses of various kinds, leading to the onset of protective brain inhibition and the hypnoid phase may suddenly open the mind in a most uncritical manner to the implantation of new ideas. This 'imprinting phase' of brain activity, as it has been called, is normally present in very young children and can be induced artificially in adults.

We have so far discussed several specific measures for dealing with anxiety – adequate sedation after traumatic events, abreaction and hypnosis. There are a number of other treatments which we can touch on briefly. Self or auto-hypnosis is coming into fashion. Hypnosis is first induced by the therapist, then the essentials of the

* Jean Martin Charcot (1825–1893). Famous French physician who pioneered psychotherapy at the Salpêtrière.

technique are acquired from him, practised under his supervision and finally employed by the patient on his own. Behaviour therapy has already been mentioned when dealing with habituation. It promises to be an important plank in the treatment of the chronic anxieties and phobias.

Systematic training in muscle relaxation was introduced by Jacobson in 1938, the hypothesis being that reduced muscle tension would lead to reduced autonomic nervous system activity. It is supposed that the anxiety state is associated with high levels of arousal, increased sympathetic activity and high levels of muscle tension. Muscle relaxation would lead to a reciprocal inhibition of the anxiety response. It may be that muscle relaxation does directly decrease anxiety or it may be that this form of relaxation is a mild self-hypnotic state, or again that inhibition of muscle tone requires inhibition of arousal and therefore lessened emotional tone. Whatever the brain mechanism, relaxation is a simple, cheap and not very time-consuming means of lessening anxiety which can be readily taught by members of a medical team, including nurses and psychologists. It may have the additional benefit of introducing rest periods during the day thus combating fatigue. The technique has been practised with success for many years in antenatal clinics and removes a considerable part of anxiety in labour.

Another form of psychotherapy which has only recently become available in this country, though it was first developed in Germany over fifty years ago by a Dr J. H. Schultz, is Autogenic Therapy.

The term 'Autogenic' literally means generated from within, and refers to two aspects of the process. Firstly, there is the basic shift from the 'Stressed State' in which people now live, to a specific, restorative, healing 'Autogenic State', which in many important ways differs from the apparently similar phase of hypnosis, and in which the brain is better able to bring about a wide range of self-regulated readjustments of many systems in the body. These periods of passive concentration on verbal stimuli, the 'Autogenic Formulae', restore the balance of the Autogenic Nervous System. The 'Stress Responses' brought about by the 'Fight and Flight' sympathetic system are reduced, and the 'Rest and Digest' actions of the parasympathetic system are increased. In this way the body moves from a state of war to one of peace.

The second aspect of 'Autogenic Therapy' which makes its title appropriate, is that the process involves the active participation of each person, and is a form of self-help. It works on the important principle that given the basic techniques, and a degree of advice and encouragement, the trainee can proceed safely to apply the method for himself between sessions with the therapist. It also avoids the transference problems seen in analysis, and can be economically applied in groups. Autogenic training is effective not only in anxiety but in many psychosomatic disorders as well.

There remain a few physical methods of combating anxiety which we have not yet mentioned. The rationale of electro-convulsive treatment is not at all clear but it is effective in severe anxiety states and depressions. Modified leucotomies are rarely carried out because of the unwillingness of surgeons to perform an irreversible operation and memories of the results of the more brutal operation of prefrontal leucotomy. The present refined operation cuts only a small number of fibres in the limbic circuit and decreases the activity of that circuit with a lessening of anxiety. Electrical stimulation of the Brain (ESB) deserves a fleeting reference. It has only been used therapeutically on rare occasions, for example in cases of schizophrenia, when electrodes were implanted into the septate region of the limbic system, but one would not be surprised if more use were made of this procedure in future, perhaps in cases of uncontrolled aggression as only minimal damage is done to the brain and no major tracts of fibres are cut.

Numerous drugs are of course used in the control of anxiety, often with justification. It is generally accepted that there is no place at all for the addictive drugs. Why, after all, exchange one illness – anxiety, for another – drug addiction. Another disturbing fact is the enormous quantity of tranquillizers and hypnotics prescribed. This might perhaps be an indication of the inadequate treatment of anxiety in its early stages, by psychotherapeutic methods. How did these millions of patients who now use tranquillizers survive in the days when these drugs were just not available? Is it that we have so much more neurosis in our midst? Are doctors making use of a time saving, readily available remedy? Is society in general failing to give the sympathy and support it might once have been prepared to give?

There must be many interwoven factors responsible for this sad state of affairs. We suspect there is a real increase in human unhappiness brought about by the hardships of industrialized urban life and we should not blind ourselves to its existence by the use of ever-increasing quantities of tranquillizers but should begin to tackle the root sources of anxiety. As this book does not pretend to be a text book of pharmacology we will leave the subject of drugs with the comment that we are grateful for the blessing of modern psychotropic drugs but should regard their overconsumption as a sign of partial failure – failure to understand the origin and nature of our pathological emotions and to exercise control by social and psychotherapeutic means. Patients should begin to ask their doctors not just to suppress their anxiety by the long-continued use of drugs but to cure them of this anxiety by a well planned programme involving social services, psychotherapy and family support.

15

*

Management of some Stress-linked Diseases

IT MAY BE OF HELP to sufferers from stress-related diseases, or indeed to their relatives, to acquire some understanding of the causal factors leading to these conditions and of the principles of treatment. Because the field is so large we have selected for discussion only some of the commoner diseases and others, which although rarer, are of particular interest. We will not attempt to give obscure technical details of drug treatment nor to be comprehensive but only to give an overall picture which will lead to better insight into the problems of management and to the involvement of the patient in his own treatment.

We have suggested that an element of chronic fatigue plays an important causative role in the rheumatic and allergic disorders and in order to avoid repetition in the following pages we recommend that in the management of these conditions, vigorous measures be taken, where necessary, to combat fatigue along the lines described in chapter nine.

Asthma

Although asthma usually presents itself as a distinct, well-recognized, entity there can be some confusion with bronchitis and no absolute separation of the two diseases is possible even with the help of objective scientific tests. We have therefore to fall back on a clinical definition of the condition such as – a partial, reversible obstruction of the airways associated with noisy expiration called wheezing. As we have pointed out in Chapter 5 three basic abnormalities characterize the asthmatic bronchial tube: spasm of the circular muscle around the tube, allergic thickening of the wall and tenacious allergic sputum which is white unless superadded infection turns it yellow or green.

The hereditary element is strong but it is not asthma that is inherited but an allergic tendency. At least two-thirds of asthmatics can trace a history of allergy in one or more of their near relatives. If both sides of the family of an affected subject give an allergic history then he is likely to suffer from some allergic manifestation early on in life such as infantile eczema, nappy rash, asthma, allergic rhinitis (nasal catarrh) or drug sensitivity. The mere fact that an infant has inherited an allergic disposition need not be too worrying to the parents. After all it may never develop asthma and even if it does, carefully planned treatment has robbed this disease of much of its historic terror. Asthma may come on at any age, and disappear at any age but it will do so most commonly at puberty. The reason why it so often departs at this period is not quite clear but by this age the purely emotional responses of childhood are being replaced by intellectually-controlled behaviour and the parent-child conflict becomes less violent. There is obviously an alteration in the quality and quantity of hormones secreted and finally the infectious diseases of childhood have been left behind. Patients may however develop their first attack in middle or old age following a severe bout of stress and, if properly managed, lose their disease shortly afterwards. Although the condition must always be taken seriously and treated with care the death rate is not alarming.

Granted a hereditary basis for the asthmatic tendency there are several triggers which can precipitate an attack. In childhood a sensitivity to some environmental allergy is common, giving rise to what is known as extrinsic asthma. The substances responsible may be pollens, housedust mite and animal furs or feathers. Moulds are less often responsible. The mite is present in nearly all households and is especially to be found in sheets and mattresses where dry human skin, its source of food, flakes off. There is therefore not the slightest shame in having these invisible creatures in one's bedroom – no one is exempt from their company. Perhaps the old German and Scandinavian habit of shaking blankets and eiderdowns out and then placing them on the window sill owes its existence to their instinctive realization that this procedure decreases the liability to asthma.

Bacterial and virus infections commonly precipitate asthma. In fact one can often trace a child's asthma to an attack of measles, whooping cough or bronchitis. The mechanism for this is not clear but there are several possibilities. The patient may be allergic to bacteria in the same way as he is to other substances such as pollens, but this is not proved. Organisms may so alter the lining of the bronchial tube that other allergic mechanisms are brought into play or they may act as simple irritants. Finally they may weaken an individual's general resistance so that he may develop an attack.

Asthma may be brought on by psychological factors. This is commonly acknowledged and it is generally held that about one third of attacks are mainly of emotional origin. There must be at least two pathways. When a patient, who knows he is allergic to certain flowers, is shown an artificial flower of the appropriate kind, he may suddenly wheeze. This must be in the nature of a conditioned reflex mediated through the autonomic nervous system and similar to the conditioned visceral reflexes brought about by Miller in animals.

More commonly psychogenic asthma is a delayed reaction to emotional stress. Psychiatrists may argue about the nature of the personality and of the traumatic events which they hold to be responsible for the attack but this does not alter the fact that whatever this might be it has to make itself felt through physical pathways which bring about the three pathological elements of asthma already described. It is not sufficient to postulate an infolding of the soft posterior part of the larger bronchial tubes in forced expiration as Joannes Groen has done, as this cannot account for the histological changes. Nor can suppressed tears be imaginatively invoked for there is no reason why the bronchial tube should take over the function of the lachrymal glands. One is forced to the conclusion that psychiatrists have not satisfactorily explained the pathological changes in asthma and have not built an acceptable bridge between emotion and the disease.

As emotional factors are acknowledged in many cases of asthma one might ask whether psychotherapy should be used. R. C. B. Aitken and his colleagues[1] at the University of Edinburgh studied sixty-eight asthmatics randomly selected from a register of diagnosed cases and, after careful psychometric tests, clinical assessment of personality traits and psychophysiological examination, came to the following conclusions. There was virtually no evidence that the distribution of psychological abnormality or psychopathology in these patients differed from that found in the general population. There was no relationship between the amount of psychopathology and the severity of the asthma. Patients with high 'psychometric emotionality' ratings benefited from attendance at a psychiatric clinic both as far as their anxiety and their asthma were concerned but this was independent of the intensity of their psychiatric treatment. It seemed logical to the authors that patients with significant psychopathology should have appropriate psychotherapy. They add that bronchospasm will probably increase anxiety (presumably because of fear of suffocation and of chronic invalidism) and that psychotherapy is likely to diminish this tendency. This seems to be a sensible and scientific approach, free from preconceived ideas, and is likely to earn the increasing support of both physicians and psychiatrists.

Asthma which arises without proved environmental allergic sensitivity is called intrinsic – stemming from within – and is probably of mixed psychological and infective origin but other, so far undiscovered factors, may play a part. Intrinsic asthma usually starts later in life, is more chronic and rather more difficult to control.

The ideas put forward in earlier sections of this book have led us to take a slightly different view of the genesis of asthma to the more commonly-held one just described. The disease is influenced for better or for worse at two levels. At the peripheral level any number of physical agents can irritate the bronchial tube depending on individual susceptibility. Challenge by allergenic material, bacteria, viruses, irritating chemicals may all bring about, singly or in combination, the pathological elements of asthma. But strangely enough, the same irritant will not always bring on an attack. There is a central factor which determines whether or not it will take place. If the central resistance is high – no asthma, if poor – an attack of moderate severity and if very low – then a severe and persistent attack. The central resistance is complex and influenced by numerous factors, some physical and some psychological. On the physical side there are debilitating illnesses such as influenza, excessive work and inadequate sleep. On the psychological side situations which create anxiety, and increase the pace of life change. Too many experiences in too short a time, whether painful or pleasurable will lower resistance. Both physical and psychological factors affect central resistance through the vehicle of chronic fatigue. There will be an exhaustion of overactive cells in the brain, which will fail to stimulate the hypothalamus sufficiently and so in turn the pituitary-adrenal axis is inadequately activated with a resultant low cortisol level, giving rise to a feeling of bodily fatigue. It is thought that this low cortisol level permits unwanted allergic inflammation and perhaps also influences the immunological mechanism to become increasingly sensitive and produce harmful antibodies.

The attack of asthma, if it is allowed to develop, is therefore brought about by a summation of factors, some peripheral and some central and treatment, if it is to be effective, must be directed at both these levels. It can readily be seen then that this is not simply a matter of prescribing a few tablets or aerosol bronchodilators but involves a detailed study of the patient and his social and family background, allergy testing and the performance of various tests of lung function.

Tablets which mimic the action of the sympathetic nervous system have long been used in the treatment of asthma. A search is made for preparations that will relieve bronchospasm without bringing about unpleasant cardio-vascular effects. Ephidrine is one of the old-fashioned kind and can be used singly or in combination with other drugs. Patients often like it in spite of its stimulant effect on the heart. Of the newer class of tablet, with minimal cardiac effect, Ventolin is useful but, given by mouth, may cause some tremor of the limbs.

For inhalation there are short-acting and long-acting aerosols. For a time they fell into disrepute, especially the former as overdosage led to cardiac complications and even death. Some of the newer short-acting aerosols and most of the longer-acting ones are relatively free of cardiac effects and, if responsibly used, are effective and safe. In mild asthma they have the advantage of acting specifically on lung tissue, allowing the use of a lower dose than would be possible by the oral route and so giving rise to fewer side effects. It must be emphasized that the number of puffs per day must be limited and that if relief is not obtained other forms of treatment must be adopted.

If the attack is severe and neither aerosol nor tablet are likely to influence it then an injection of Adrenaline under the skin can be dramatically useful. The drug should never be given into a vein or be administered by the patient himself.

Drugs such as Choledyl or Aminophylline also bring about

relaxation of bronchial tubes. When given by mouth they are harmless and gently effective. Indeed in one trial they were found to be as effective as Intal (see below) but this claim may be somewhat exaggerated. These drugs may be given by venous route in an emergency under expert medical care, often with prompt relief.

Until the advent of Intal cortico-steroids were regarded as the wonder drugs of asthma. They are still highly regarded but used with caution and restraint as side effects and complications can be common and serious. The pituitary hormone ACTH is not itself a steroid but stimulates the adrenal cortex to produce cortisol. It is ineffective by mouth and must be given by injection. It has a place in the treatment of some cases of severe, persistent asthma not responding to simpler measures. The advantages it has over steroids are firstly, that it does not suppress the adrenal cortex and secondly, that it does not inhibit growth in children. But it has disadvantages of its own. It will induce sluggishness of the pituitary gland itself, it has the same range of unwanted side effects as the steroids and, as the naturally occurring product is of animal origin, it may bring about an allergic response and become ineffective. Finally if the adrenal gland is already wasted from previous use of steroids then there will be a false sense of security, ACTH will fail to stimulate the adrenal cortex and the attack will worsen. The newer, synthetic corticotrophic hormones have the same properties as naturally occurring ACTH but allergic reactions are fewer.

Cortisone, one of the earliest adrenal steroids to be produced commercially is not now used in asthma except by injection. It has been replaced by a number of similar, yet more powerful synthetic drugs, with fewer side effects, like prednisone. In spite of the undoubted value of these cortico-steroids we should not rush into their use for they have a long list of serious side effects. We have been unable to detach the anti-allergic and anti-inflammatory properties from their other properties and so continued use may cause wasting of the adrenal glands, high blood pressure, diabetes, peptic ulcer, weakness of bone and muscle and so on. The aim therefore is to use an adequate dose of cortico-steroids for short periods only and avoid maintenance treatment wherever possible. Another strategy is to use alternative day treatment which allows the adrenal gland to function normally one day in two and lessens the likelihood of its wasting.

If the patient is very distressed and oral prednisone, which takes four or more hours to act, is considered to be inadequate, then an injection of cortisol into a vein is very helpful.

Recently an aerosol cortico-steroid, Becotide, has been developed which acts directly on lung tissue, is hardly absorbed into the blood stream and therefore gives rise to negligible generalized side effects. It is a most useful drug provided the tubes are open enough for the mist to reach the bronchioles. There is a minor disadvantage in that a small proportion of patients will develop a fungal infection of the upper respiratory tract and become hoarse. The aerosol will allow many patients who would otherwise have had to be on maintenance doses of oral steroids to manage without them and so be much less at risk from major side effects. Patients should realize that the aerosol is of a different nature to the ones which have adrenaline-like properties and must be taken at constant and only gradually adjusted doses.

We come to Intal (Cromoglycate) which represents a major advance in treatment. It acts at the level of the smaller bronchial tubes where it suppresses the liberation of histamine and its companions which induce the allergic reaction. It is therefore prophylactic or preventive and cannot be used to abort an attack already in being. It has been found effective in most cases of extrinsic, in some cases of intrinsic and in exercise induced asthma. Again the bronchial tubes must be clear to allow penetration of the powder through an ingenious apparatus looking like a jet engine. It can be used if the attacks do not respond to adrenaline-like drugs. It may obviate the need for steroids in the severer cases but sometimes only succeeds in reducing the dose of steroid required and this is a great gain. There are no appreciable side effects. One usually starts with four capsules per day and then slowly decreases to the minimum dose required. Fluctuation in dosage should be avoided.

Antibiotics have an important place in asthma. Even patients with predominantly extrinsic asthma will, from time to time, have attacks brought on by infection. If one follows patients through the years then one will see allergic asthma subsiding to be replaced more and more by infective asthma and bronchitis. The aim is not only to rid the patient of asthma but to leave him with undamaged lungs. So, whenever there is an infective element a case can be made out for the use of antibiotics in addition to drugs for the relief of spasm. The argument is sometimes advanced that the attack has been precipitated by a viral infection which is not amenable to antibiotics and so none need be given. The fallacy here is that it is difficult to distinguish between viral and bacterial symptoms, and, in any case, bacterial infection will so often complicate a viral onset.

The allergic element in asthma may be dealt with in two main ways. Firstly, by environmental control, the offending substance such as pollens, feathers or house dust being avoided as far as practical or, where possible, removed from the vicinity of the patient. Secondly, where history and allergy testing are in agreement and the material cannot readily be avoided, then desensitization or hyposensitization (which is more correct) can be employed through a course of injections. This method is not often called for, but it can, at times, be extremely effective especially if a single substance such as housedust mite is largely responsible or a well-defined small group such as grass pollens.

Having decided that the personality and experiences of the patient are not specific there can be no standard psychiatric approach but each case is assessed for its mental component and treatment tailored accordingly. Some cases are entirely healthy from the psychological angle, having robust personalities and no significant emotional problems, others only have anxiety as a result of asthma. The former need no psychotherapy while the latter need only good general treatment and reassurance. Where the emotional component is marked then a whole range of psychotherapy is applicable from mild supportive measures to psychoanalysis. The choice of treatment depends on the complexity of the psychopathology, the skills of the GP and of the available consultants. It rests not on the diagnosis of asthma but on the type of neurosis which is present in any particular case.

The aim of psychotherapy is an improvement of personality function on a broad front. It should give insight into the factors which can trigger attacks (after all understanding and predictability decrease fear). Wherever possible interpersonal relationships should be improved and friction lessened. Specific neuroses should be treated and attempts should be made to reduce the patient's sensitivity and vulnerability. His burden of anxiety and fear should be explored and mitigated. Decreased wastage of emotional energy should be encouraged and a well-founded optimistic approach to his illness fostered. Antidepressants, tranquillizers and mild hypnotics may all at times have a place in treatment, preferably on a short term basis.

A major means of restoring health and therefore counteracting asthma is to improve the quality and quantity of sleep. Sleep will have been impaired and reduced by the attack itself or by a concomitant depression. A great deal of energy is used in the course of an attack and anxiety may sap energy stores still further. Sleep must be regarded as the logical antidote. The need for extra sleep should therefore be carefully explained to the patient and parent. The amount required is that which will counteract and abolish fatigue and the quality that of natural, undrugged sleep but if this will not come spontaneously then a mild hypnotic is justified which will not interfere with dream sleep or depress respiration. An afternoon rest, if it can be fitted in, is highly desirable. Little children will readily take advice from a friendly doctor whereas they might pay no attention at all to their parents.

Exercise has two opposing effects. On the one hand it is beneficial as it improves general health, creates self-confidence and boosts the efficiency of the musculature and cardiovascular system. There is also evidence that it increases the size of the adrenal cortex and permits a greater production of cortisol in times of stress. On the other hand exercise may itself precipitate asthma. The wise course of action is therefore to allow and even encourage exercise with two provisos. First the patient must stop at once if wheezing comes on even if in the middle of a competitive game and secondly, if Intal can be shown to be of value in his particular case, he should take it prior to exercise. It goes without saying that he should not even think of exercise if he is already wheezy or if he is tired. Many asthmatics are good at games and get great pleasure out of them. This says a lot for the efficiency of treatment these days.

The treatment of asthma can be left on a cheerful note. We have a reasonable understanding of the pathology of the disease and of the numerous factors which lead to it. We have a wide and increasingly effective range of drugs and so we can give the majority of patients a reassurance that they will be able to lead normal and unhampered lives. In our experience the outlook is only poor where irremovable stress factors exist such as a positive hatred and irreconcilable conflict between firmly linked relatives.

Hay Fever

If asthma conjures up to the patient the image of a turbulent ocean which he and his physician must navigate with great skill then hay fever is, by comparison, a calm lake to be crossed with relative ease – a nuisance rather than a threat. It is obviously seasonal and the result of an allergy to pollens of various kinds, but one cannot dismiss the stress factor altogether. The question must be posed – why does one subject of an allergic disposition develop it and not another and why should he do so at that particular time of his life? We cannot be certain about the answer but it seems to us most likely that the onset is related to stress, fatigue and a prolonged exposure to high levels of pollen and that a central factor of resistance and susceptibility is at play as we have surmised in asthma.

The condition must be distinguished from allergic, but non-seasonal, rhinitis in which the culprit may be the house-dust mite and from non-allergic all-the-year-round rhinitis which is usually called vasomotor rhinitis and may be triggered off by changes in temperature or by fatigue. If the mite should be responsible then there may be mild symptoms all the year round with perhaps a peak in the winter months from about October to February. It is just as well to have the diagnosis confirmed by a competent allergist before embarking on treatment which may last two or three years or even a lifetime. The most common tests to be carried out are prick tests on the skin. Occasionally direct provocation tests on the lining of the nose are needed.

There are several aspects to treatment. Advice is sometimes given to avoid pollens by staying away from the countryside and parks or by closing windows at night. This seems too high a price to pay and we would not recommend it except in very resistant cases and when the published pollen count is very high.

Antihistamines are of great help to the majority of patients both in relieving catarrh and eye symptoms. Some individuals do not become drowsy when given these drugs and they do best. In those that do become sleepy a large dose, in long-acting form, can be given at bedtime and smaller, short acting, doses as needed by day, or else a less soporific antihistamine can be chosen for day time use.

Rynacrom, similar to Intal, is useful but very expensive. Its use is justified in those that are intolerant of, or unresponsive to, antihistamines and is then given as a powder for insufflation with a special apparatus or in the form of a spray. It must be employed regularly and sufficiently frequently to start with and decreased gradually to the minimum required.

Local steroids, in the form of a Beconase spray, are effective, as is the case in asthma. One would not, however, have recourse to them unless both antihistamines and Rynacrom have failed. It is possible that long term use could cause thinning of the lining of the nasal passages.

If symptoms are not controlled by these measures, or if pollen asthma co-exists then a course of desensitization by injections can be considered. These should be carried out with due precautions against possible, but rare, allergic reactions. For example, the patient must be prepared to stay in the surgery after the injection for a twenty minute period of observation. Arrangements for the injection must be made well in advance of the hay fever season, say in January and the first injection is usually given in late February. To achieve any lasting benefit courses will need to be given yearly for some three years. Patients would be unwise to expect a one hundred per cent relief, but should be satisfied with something in the order of seventy-five per cent. Antihistamines or other measures may still be required at peak pollen periods.

Nothing is ever said about general measures in the treatment of hay fever but, as we have already mentioned, there is surely a central factor of resistance which must be taken into account and therefore steps should be taken to increase the general level of health, by physical and psychological means, similar to those advocated in asthma; but in view of the lesser severity of symptoms these steps need not be so energetic.

The Rheumatic Diseases

There is a world of difference between, let us say, rheumatic fever, rheumatoid arthritis, osteo-arthritis and lumbago but there are also many common characteristics which link them together. Firstly, they all affect some elements of 'connective tissue' which embraces ligaments, joint linings, tendons, discs, cartilage, heart valves, and the deeper portions of the skin. Secondly, there is a wide overlap of symptoms and clinical findings. For example, rheumatic nodules are found in rheumatic fever and rheumatoid arthritis; inflamed joints are present in many of these illnesses even where spinal symptoms predominate. Thirdly, there is evidence of an autoimmune phenomenon in the majority of these conditions. Fourthly, and more speculatively, there is the element of stress and chronic fatigue which appears to be shared by them all. We are therefore justified in considering the rheumatic problems as a group and it also follows that treatment of the separate conditions will contain a core of similarity.

Rheumatoid Arthritis

The causes of rheumatoid arthritis have already been referred to in the chapters on psychosomatic disease and fatigue. There appears to be a thread of heredity which is not very strong. Most doctors will agree that stress is an ingredient and our previous discussion leans towards non-specific psychological factors as opposed to specific personality and experience in the stress situation. A modern suspicion is that a virus or bacteria may so alter joint tissue as to initiate an autoimmune process. That is antibodies will be formed which attack the lining of the joints. The disease is a common one and will affect some two to three per cent of the adult population, women being at greater risk.

Treatment is complex and requires subtle decisions as to the best approach. It is imperative to catch the disease early, hold a watching brief and intervene energetically if there is any evidence of deterioration. The clinical picture of rheumatoid arthritis is different to that of simple osteo-arthritis and, where the former is suspected, a greater effort should be made as it is potentially so much more crippling.

To judge progress it is advisable to arrange a base line of simple blood tests and one or two X-rays of affected joints. It is probable that in the early stages 'rheumatoid factor' will be absent and the red cell sedimentation rate will be only slightly raised. X-rays are unlikely to show any erosion of bone. So much the better. Simple clinical assessment of some of the affected joints will help to establish the degree of involvement.

As in the case of asthma, the whole person will need to be considered, not just his painful points. His personality and traumatic personal experiences should be explored and this process can be most rewarding.

The patient is given as full an explanation as possible of the contributory causes to his illness and the probable mechanism of their action, and any psychological or physical strain is dealt with as appropriate. If the illness is not rapidly and effectively controlled at an early stage then it will pay handsome dividends to tackle it more energetically. It is the central resistance which needs building up by adequate rest, controlled exercise, hospital or sanatorium admission where required, relief from psychological stress within the family and work milieu, and protection from financial strain. The patients may require a sheltered convalescence and should not return to full duties till the disease process can be shown to have abated.

There is a wide choice of drugs which lies between various aspirin preparations, a number of other, newer anti-inflammatory drugs, gold, cortico-steroids, and penicillamine. Aspirin and the anti-inflammatory drugs are relatively safe while the others are potentially harmful and need careful supervision by an experienced rheumatologist. The latter drugs are reserved for the more serious and progressive type of disease where their benefits outweigh their dangers. Aspirin is underrated by most patients. It is a powerful antirheumatic drug whose effectiveness can be seen when it is used in acute rheumatic fever. The disadvantage of aspirin – its tendency to irritate the lining of the stomach and cause minor bleeding – can be overcome by using an enteric-coated preparation which ensures that it does not become active until it reaches the small intestine, or by use of such drugs as Palaprin or Benoral which, although expensive, do not irritate the stomach.

The newer anti-inflammatory drugs which include Butazolidin, Brufen and Indocid are perhaps marginally more effective than aspirin and, if this has not been well tolerated, then the doctor can choose a preparation out of this group which will suit his particular patient. They are not free from side effects but these tend to be minor. Butazolidin should be used with greater care than some of the others as it occasionally does harm to the bone marrow. Indocid is less toxic but may cause some dyspepsia. Brufen is very well tolerated though, perhaps, less powerful.

Gold has been in and out of favour for many years. The present generally-accepted view is that it can be very effective but its use must be carefully supervised as it may damage kidneys, bone marrow and skin and courses should perhaps be maintained far longer than previously thought necessary.

As in the case of other chronic illnesses such as asthma corticosteroids should be avoided except for short-term use. Their long-term side effects are intolerable. Injection of cortisone into the joint itself would appear to be a logical, useful and harmless process but experience has shown that it is of limited value especially in weight-bearing joints where it can cause an acceleration of wear and tear of the cartilaginous surfaces.

The importance of physiotherapy has decreased because of the greater efficiency of drug treatment and our increased understanding of the role of psychological and social factors but nevertheless it still plays a useful part in immobilizing acutely inflamed joints by various forms of splinting and in combating pain. Later it is called upon to restore mobility, to prevent deformity of joints and disuse wasting of muscles.

The Social Services can provide many mechanical aids to help patients with weakness or deformity so as to allow them to work in their own homes or in sheltered occupations outside. They can also act as a buffer between the patient and his financial obligations and they can provide home helps, meals on wheels and numerous other helpful services.

A great deal can be accomplished by carefully-considered surgical intervention. Perhaps the most significant contribution of surgery is in restoring movement to severely destroyed, deformed and unstable joints or in the relief of intolerable pain but some claim is made that synovectomy (the removal of inflamed synovial membrane or joint lining) can arrest the progress of the disease in the affected joint and, if all else fails, then this might be undertaken.

There was a vogue in the 1950s for the correction of a raised blood pressure by surgical removal of parts of the sympathetic nervous system. But this became obsolete with the development of adequate drug treatment. It may be that surgical treatment of rheumatoid joints is in such a historical phase and will become largely unnecessary with improved understanding of the disease and better medical treatment.

OSTEO-ARTHRITIS (OA)

Some of the predisposing factors to this common degenerative condition which affects mainly the larger joints such as hips and knees but does not entirely spare the smaller joints, are:– A mild hereditary element, obesity, advancing years, trauma and excessive use in work and sport. Well over half the population above the age of fifty will suffer from it.

Treatment of osteo-arthritis is similar in many respects to that of chronic rheumatoid arthritis. Obesity must be prevented at all costs as increased weight will result in increased trauma to the weight-bearing joints. Our image of health and personal attractiveness is slowly changing from that of the portly male and buxom female of Victorian times to the slim figure of today and this will not only cut our food import bills but also reduce the incidence of osteo-arthritis. The slogan should be 'slim is beautiful'.

Occupations and sports which lead to excessive trauma and arthritis should be carefully supervised. Where physical stress is excessive mechanical aids might be called upon. Protective pads could be worn over exposed points. For instance the knee might be shielded where work is done in the kneeling position. Longer rest periods might be organized between shifts. It is probably unwise to participate in an active, competitive game unless one is well rested and free from joint pain. A slightly damaged joint may be further damaged with unpleasant long term consequences. Fatigue prior to the game may well indicate a lack of facility for repair of damaged joints.

Although there is no evidence of inflammation in the majority of affected joints and the sedimentation rate is usually normal, this cannot be categorically ruled out and there is some overlap between rheumatoid arthritis and OA. In fact OA frequently complicates rheumatoid arthritis. In view of this anti-inflammatory drugs are often more appropriate than simple analgesic drugs. In other words one would seek to control not only pain but also inflammation and would use various preparations of aspirin and drugs like Brufen and Indocid in preference to simple painkilling drugs like Paracetemol or Distalgesic, although the latter can be used in addition to anti-inflammatory drugs. Cortico-steroids are rarely used and then only by injection into a joint. Physiotherapy and surgery are brought in on the same principles as in rheumatoid arthritis.

ACUTE RHEUMATIC FEVER

This condition is now fortunately extremely rare and the decline in its incidence has taken place over the past thirty years, in fact since the advent of Penicillin. In its severe form it can lead to distortion of the valves of the heart with serious cardiac invalidism so that its near eradication is a triumph of medicine and evidence also of improved living standards. The only point to be made is that General Practitioners have very wisely given Penicillin, since it became available, for tonsillitis, paying no attention to words of caution from some specialists who argued that this was unnecessary. The streptococcus, which plays an essential role in the genesis of rheumatic fever, is thus killed off and the disease averted. Common sense has prevailed over 'scientific' hesitations.

POLYMYALGIA RHEUMATICA (Otherwise – painful muscles of rheumatic origin)

This is a fascinating condition affecting elderly people. At one time the disease was ill-understood and many of these old folk were considered to be neurotic or depressed. Gradually it became clear that they were suffering from a serious complaint associated with the inflammation of joints and soft tissues, a very high sedimentation rate, weight loss and general debility, and that there was some degree of overlap with an even more serious condition called temporal arteritis in which the arteries at the sides of the forehead were inflamed, and where vision could be lost through involvement of the retinal arteries. So at last the old people got the treatment they needed which, as can be guessed, is cortico-steroids.

The following sad case emphasizes the role of stress in the origin of this complaint. An old man was living happily in retirement with his wife. One evening she collapsed while dancing with him and died shortly afterwards of an acute heart attack. He pretended that he had adjusted himself to his bereavement but this was not really so and after a few weeks he developed polymyalgia rheumatica with severe pain and morning stiffness. He responded to steroids but never regained complete health.

CERVICAL SPONDYLOSIS, LUMBAGO AND SCIATICA

Pain in the neck and in the lower back is, as everyone knows, extremely common and few escape it at some time in their lives. The spinal cord runs in a long canal behind the bodies of the vertebrae and coming off the cord are nerves which pass to the limbs and trunk. Compression of these nerves at different levels

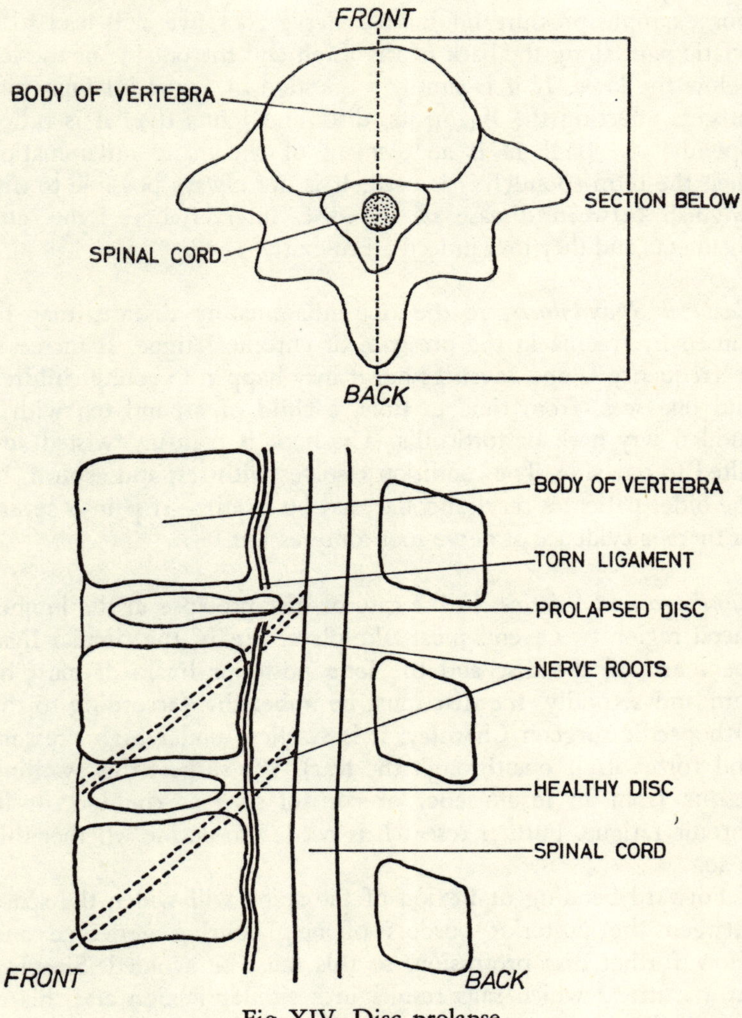

Fig XIV. Disc prolapse

by prolapsed discs or narrowing of the apertures between the vertebrae, through which they have to pass, leads to pain referred to various parts such as the back of the skull, the shoulder girdle and upper limbs, the trunk and lower limbs as the case may be. For example pressure on lumbar nerve root five will lead to a sciatic pain along the back of the thigh and the outside of the leg below the knee. If it is simply a question of a non-inflammatory process affecting the ligaments, discs and joints then it is called Spondylosis. If there is an element of rheumatic inflammation then the term spondylitis is used. It is not always possible to distinguish between disease of the disc, intervertebral joints and ligaments and they may indeed all co-exist.

Cervical Spondylosis, ie the non-inflammatory disease, may be caused by trauma in the presence of chronic fatigue. It increases in frequency as age advances but it may happen to young children and one sees, from time to time, a child of around ten with a sudden wry neck or torticollis. The neck is painful, twisted and tilted to one side. The condition resolves with rest and aspirin. In the older patient a cervical collar may be required if pain is severe or there is evidence of nerve root compression.

Lumbago and Sciatica. In the case of disc prolapse in the lumbosacral region two events must take place. Firstly, the circular ligament around the disc and the long posterior ligament must be torn and secondly, the disc must be unhealthy (according to the orthopaedic surgeon Charnley, it is swollen, under high pressure and forces itself out through the tear). We suspect this swelling results from an insufficiency of cortisol such as could occur in chronic fatigue. Further research is needed to decide whether this is so.

Forward bending or flexion of the spine will widen the space between the posterior borders of neighbouring vertebrae and allow further disc protrusion, so this must be avoided. Sleeping on a mattress which sags results in a similar flexion and this is remedied by placing a piece of hardboard approximately five feet by three feet under the mattress. Carrying a heavy weight will put grea[illegible]ssure on the disc and squeeze it out through the already [illegible]nents, so weight carrying is prohibited while there is pain. [illegible]t is necessary for two reasons. First, to counteract chronic fatigue and second, to take the weight of the body off the affected disc space. Lying in bed may appear to aggravate pain but a comfortable position, if need be in flexion, can usually be found. Later it will become possible to straighten out the spine and lie flat on the back. Bed rest need not and cannot be absolute. The patient will prefer in most cases to get up to toilet and eat his meals in a sitting position out of bed. Indeed attempts to eat in bed may so flex the spine as to be counter productive.

When pain has largely settled extension exercises may help to strengthen the muscles of the spine and encourage correct posture. Flexion exercises must of course be carefully avoided. Physiotherapy does not play a significant role in lumbago. Some hospitals still indulge in stretching the spine with a machine which resembles an Elizabethan rack. A harness is attached above and below the disc lesion and the two are gradually pulled apart. It does little harm but equally little good. (Stretching of the cervical spine on the other hand, in cases where nerve root pressure makes this desirable, seems to be more effective.) Heat, massage and exercises have a marginal influence on progress, the disc is after all very deeply placed.

The value of manipulation is in dispute. Its adherents claim that it will either bring the disc back into its rightful place – which seems to be a tall order as the button-like shape projects through a slit in the posterior ligament; one cannot imagine how that button will return through its slit – or, that the disc will be extruded and fall harmlessly into the fluid space around the spinal cord. Here again this could happen or matters could be made worse by partial extrusion and increased pressure on the sciatic nerve. One has come across cases in which the patient has gone to the manipulator with lumbago and has left him with both lumbago and an unwanted present – sciatica. Some cases do benefit, but it is difficult to know in advance who will improve and who deteriorate. As a matter of principle therefore it might be wise to avoid manipulation in most cases until one can be satisfied by controlled research that it has a useful role. If, in spite of discussion, the patient demands a manipulation then it is suggested that a medically qualified specialist should be used who will understand the dangers and limitations of the procedure.

If we turn back for a moment to consider manipulation of the cervical spine then one would be even more insistent on a medically qualified manipulator, for here there is increased danger of serious consequences, especially if there is an element of rheumatoid arthritis of the neck when unskilled manipulation can result in damage to the long nerve tracts in the spinal cord with partial paralysis of the limbs.

Painkilling drugs give partial relief, but obviously drugs of addiction should be avoided. Surgical corsets with steel supports are supplied and worn for intractable pain. By restricting movement, especially flexion, they may be helpful but long term use, which will probably cause disuse wasting of some of the spinal muscles, is not recommended.

X-rays using contrast media may show up a prolapsed disc and this can be removed surgically if medical measures have failed. In some cases operation allows the patient to return to manual labour, involving bending and lifting but this is not always the case and recurrence of pain may take place, possibly as a result of protrusion of a neighbouring disc. In other words the operation is often worthwhile but success cannot be guaranteed.

Persistent lumbago and sciatica are often linked with persistent psychological and physical stress. When, for example, the patient is involved in a serious marital problem which he cannot resolve, the continuous mental turmoil leads to chronic fatigue and loss of powers of repair to injured tissues. Numerous cases of this kind have been observed. They will only settle when the trauma of marital breakdown has been left behind. The disc sufferer may need psychotherapy or in appropriate cases, marriage guidance. Simple chronic fatigue, not associated with unhappiness, may precipitate disc protrusion but recovery proceeds rapidly once fatigue is counteracted by sufficient sleep. The French writer Ernest Feydeau, seems to have had insight into this condition. In his mid-nineteenth century play *Le Dindon*, he describes a character with Don Juan tendencies, who was at one time desperately in love with a married woman, but she resisted his advances and remained virtuous. However, one day when she had quarrelled with her husband, she decided to pay an amorous visit to her adoring friend only to find him hobbling about like an old man, crippled with lumbago (due to an excess of recent adventures) and he was only able to murmur in disappointment, resignation and sadness, 'Ah Lucienne!', but the visit remained a platonic one and virtue inadvertently triumphed.

ANKYLOSING SPONDYLITIS

A most important discovery was made in 1973 regarding hereditary factors in ankylosing spondylitis and associated rheumatic diseases. For a long time it has been known that there were antigens on the surface of all body cells which explained the rejection of grafts of various tissues from one donor to another if the tissues were not correctly matched. It is convenient to type these antigens using human leucocytes and consequently the antigens have come to be known as HL–A antigens. The inheritance of these antigens is associated with specific immune responses. By investigating the antigenic inheritance of patients with specific diseases it has become clear that certain rheumatic conditions and allergies are linked with specific HL–A antigens. Over ninety per cent of patients with ankylosing spondylitis inherit the antigen HL–A27 as opposed to only seven per cent of the general population. A similar high incidence of HL–A27 is found in patients suffering from psoriasis, ulcerative colitis and Crohn's disease complicated by ankylosing spondylitis. This work has established beyond doubt that certain, not very common, forms of rheumatism are partly inherited and leads one to believe that a hereditary element of some kind may be found in other forms of rheumatism. However only a small proportion of people who inherit this particular antigen will in fact develop an ankylosing spondylitis (about ten per cent of the men and three per cent of the women) so that environmental factors, perhaps of infection or stress, enter into the equation and determine the presence or absence of the disease.

Briefly, ankylosing spondylitis is characterized by a rheumatic inflammation of intervertebral joints leading to ossification of ligaments (showing on X-ray as a bamboo spine) and some degree of immobility of the spine and rib cage, as the posterior ends of the ribs are attached to the spine.

As to treatment genetic counselling will no doubt play a part in prevention. As the disease is not so common we will not go into the relative merits of analgesics, anti-inflammatory drugs, X-ray treatment and cortico-steroids except to say that the last two measures have largely fallen into disrepute because of side effects. It is essential not to indulge in too much bed rest in this condition so as to avoid loss of mobility of the spine and rib cage. With care the patient should retain a satisfactory posture and adequate movement of spine and chest to permit limited work and a reasonable enjoyment of life.

CARPAL TUNNEL SYNDROME

A small nerve at the front of the wrist called the median nerve is sometimes compressed in its journey through the carpal tunnel by rheumatic processes in the tunnel or nerve sheath and this leads to early morning pain, tingling and numbness in the fingers supplied by the nerve – the three and a half outer fingers if the palm is facing forwards. There may also be some pain in the forearm. It is a fairly common condition in pregnancy and in rheumatoid arthritis but may occur independently in patients, usually women, suffering from chronic fatigue.

Treatment consists in relieving pain with analgesic tablets and at times the use of comfortable night splints. A local injection of cortisone is often very effective and, if all else fails, surgical decompression, which is quite a minor procedure, may be undertaken.

FROZEN SHOULDER

By no means all painful and stiff shoulders are 'frozen' shoulders, nevertheless it is a very common condition and implies a severe inflammation of the capsule of the joint with significant limitation of movement. It may follow injury or forced immobility of the joint and sometimes even painful conditions in the chest such as a coronary thrombosis. It is more common in women and in the older age groups and, again, is probably associated with stress and fatigue.

Anti-inflammatory drugs such as Brufen and Indocid are of some help in treatment. To maintain the maximum amount of movement it is wise to carry out gentle active and passive exercises, increasing in range as the condition becomes less painful. Often the patient needs to be referred to an expert for local injections of cortisone.

TENNIS ELBOW AND SIMILAR CONDITIONS

Especially vulnerable to the rheumatic process are areas where tendons and muscles are inserted into bone. Tennis elbow is an example. Here the forearm muscles inserted into the outer aspect of the lower end of the humerus are affected. Tennis is rarely the cause – housework and carrying of shopping baskets being far more likely precipitants.

Treatment resembles that for 'frozen shoulder'. Anti-inflammatory tablets are given, the joint is at first partly rested, and injections of cortisone are very effective.

16

*

Management of Stress-Linked Diseases

Hypertension (High Blood Pressure)

HYPERTENSION MAY BE PRIMARY, and of uncertain origin, or secondary to disease of kidneys, of endocrine glands or to other known factors. The primary disease is thought to be psychosomatic in nature but this is not proven. There is no doubt that in heightened emotion whether pleasant or unpleasant, a rise in adrenaline and noradrenaline secretion takes place and that there will be a concomitant, transient rise of pulse rate and blood pressure. There is also no doubt that in conditions of work stress the blood pressure rises. What is not known is whether these episodes of hypertension will eventually develop into sustained hypertension. James Henry and his co-workers[1] were able to so alter the social environment of mice as to produce a prolonged rise in systolic blood pressure. This work suggests that appropriate psycho-social stimuli could bring about a sustained hypertension in human beings. For the moment we can only assume that the condition is due to a combination of several factors such as heredity, the level of salt intake, personality and stressful psychosocial stimuli.

The vital point about hypertension is that, on a statistical basis available to Life Insurance Companies, there is an increasing risk to life with each rise of BP above normal. For example, if we take men aged forty-five those with a normal BP of 120/80 will have a life expectancy of thirty-two years, while if the BP is 150/100 it falls to 20.5 years, ie a tremendous loss of 11.5 years. This drop of life expectancy is due to strokes, heart disease and arterial complications of all kinds. Unfortunately many patients with hypertension are symptom-free and do not report to their doctors and many with known hypertension are somewhat unwilling to accept treatment, which might involve some side effects, as they feel so well.

In view of these considerations the treatment of hypertension will need to be many sided. A Health Education Campaign should be mounted to explain the dangers of undiagnosed hypertension to the public at large and encourage it to attend for routine screening at the GP's surgery or at Welfare Clinics (eg Well Woman's Clinic). There are already several arrangements for this and details can be obtained from the Department of Health.

Hypertension cannot normally be diagnosed at one session as blood pressure varies from moment to moment and fluctuates with mood. So whereas a normal reading is reassuring, a high reading needs review. If the hypertension is mild the necessary investigations can usually be carried out by the GP and treatment be initiated there and then. If severe, then fuller investigations need to be carried out at hospital. Very rarely a definite cause amenable to surgery, can be found and corrected; for example narrowing of a section of the aorta, the main artery leading from the heart, or one sided disease of a kidney. More usually, no cause is found, the condition is labelled primary or idiopathic, and symptomatic medical treatment is given.

Patients should not be too worried about side effects of drugs. There are many mild, harmless agents which have almost no side effects yet are useful in the less severe forms of hypertension. Even when treating the more severe forms it should be possible to find drugs which do not produce faintness on standing and which do not induce impotence in the male. We would agree with the patient that the treatment must not be more unpleasant than the disease and it should be possible for most cases to be treated with drugs which do not give rise to unacceptable side effects. β Blockers like Trasicor and Inderal are especially valuable where anxiety, rapid pulse or angina co-exist.

There have now been several trials of relaxation in the treatment of hypertension, some based on natural physiological methods, others achieved with the help of Yoga and/or Biofeedback techniques,[2] that is techniques in which biological information is fed back to the subject during the period of relaxation to help him to achieve his goal. It has been shown that even with simple twice daily, non-cultic (not involving Yoga or other cult) relaxation a reasonable fall of BP can be achieved. Autogenic training is another useful means of obtaining the same effect. In mild forms of hypertension this may be all that is required while in the severe forms it may decrease the need for blood pressure lowering drugs.

Patients with hypertension and therefore possibly damaged arteries are well advised to take care of their diets from two points of view. Firstly, if they are obese they should aim to reduce weight by total calorie reduction to their optimum level and secondly, they should pursue a low animal fat diet. Both measures will lower the level of blood fats and help to safeguard the arterial system.

Atherosclerosis (Including *Angina, Strokes* and *Peripheral Artery Disease*)

Atheroma is a Greek word meaning porridge and Atherosclerosis is a term applied to medium-sized and larger arteries signifying thickening, narrowing and deformity of these arteries partly by deposition, in plaques, of a porridgy material composed mainly of cholesterol crystals. There are several processes which contribute to this state of affairs. Cholesterol can seep through the delicate inner lining of an artery and be deposited in its wall if the blood cholesterol is raised and if the pressure in the artery is high. This probably also applies to Triglycerides. Clots, or thrombi, can be formed over damaged portions of arterial lining to bulge into the lumen, or interior, of the artery and fatty material can be deposited into these thrombi as they become mature. Hypertension can aggravate the situation by causing a reactive thickening of the vessel wall and by increasing seepage of fatty material through the lining.

We need not discuss separately the treatment of the main condition in which the predominant culprit is Atherosclerosis, ie angina and coronary thrombosis (the former due to partial obstruction of the blood flow in the coronary, or heart arteries and the latter usually to total obstruction); strokes due to insufficient blood flow in the cerebral arteries or haemorrhage through a vessel wall; and Intermittent Claudication (limping) caused by a deficiency of blood supply to the legs. As atherosclerosis is the fundamental common denominator it is only necessary to discuss general measures of value in that condition.

Our present evidence to incriminate emotional factors in the genesis of atherosclerosis is building up but the relationship has, admittedly, not been proved. The same applies to diet. As far as the former proposition is concerned we know that blood fats are raised in situations of fear and anger and that in our prevailing culture these fats are not used as sources of energy (as they would be in the natural state of flight or fight) but accumulate for a time in the bloodstream where they can be harmful. We know that in large populations a high level of blood cholesterol is linked with a high level of arterial disease. We therefore suspect that transient peaks of blood fats can result in deposition of cholesterol in the artery wall.

Another speculation not often referred to, is the role of fear in the clotting mechanism. When animals meet in physical conflict they must have provision for the stemming of blood loss and this is, in fact, the case. Fear and anger increase the speed of clotting and this can be demonstrated in patients about to undergo electro-convulsive treatment, which is to them a frightening prospect. On this basis we must expect clotting to take place, more readily in diseased blood vessels, when we are in a state of fear or anger and there is some evidence that this is so.

As atherosclerosis is built up insidiously over several decades starting in childhood it should be a matter of principle in every household that the diet should not be excessive in total calories – as this in itself can result in high triglyceride blood levels – and that there should be some limitation to the animal fat content.

Obesity is an additional hazard to the atherosclerotic patient and should be brought under control preferably by dietary means. Smoking brings about a rise in blood adrenaline and noradrenaline and blood fats and whether this explains its effect on the vascular system or whether additional unpleasant mechanisms are at play, it is a dangerous pastime and should be totally given up by the atherosclerotic patient.

Lack of exercise is certainly responsible for much morbidity in the vascular sphere. Professor Morris and his colleagues demonstrated many years ago that bus drivers were far more liable to coronary heart disease than Clippies who climbed up and down the steps of their buses hundreds of times a day. This theory has been substantiated again and again leaving no doubt about the value of exercise in the prevention of coronary heart disease. As a matter of general principle then, we should be a nation of players, gardeners, walkers and cyclers rather than watchers, sitters and car drivers. Even after a coronary attack it is wise to undertake regular, moderately strenuous exercise, within the capacity of the heart, as soon as possible as this will go a long way to prevention of a recurrence. (*F/40: Fitness in forty minutes per week– might be a useful guide.*)[3]

There are several non-dietary means of lowering blood fats. If triglycerides are high, and this can be a familial matter, then Atromid S (clofibrate) is useful. If cholesterol levels are high either Atromid S or Questran (cholestyramine) can be used, the latter acting by getting rid of materials needed for fat absorption. Whether diet alone or one of these drugs in addition should be used must be left to the physician in charge. Present evidence on the value of clofibrate after an attack of coronary thrombosis is not conclusive but in the stage of angina it seems to have a definite protective effect.

Hypertension is definitely a factor in aggravating atherosclerosis and precipitating the three major complications. There is some hesitation in reducing blood flow in already narrowed and damaged arteries, but, provided the reduction of pressure is not too steep, it will be extremely worthwhile.

Finally we come to the treatment of psychological factors. Bearing in mind the increased risk of thrombosis in combat situations which we have already discussed and the findings of Peter Taggart and Carruthers of raised adrenaline and some blood fats in public speakers there seems to be some justification for an attempt at the control of emotions in people at risk.

To reinforce the theoretical evidence for a link between emotions and arterial disease we would like to recall three illustrative cases – obviously not of statistical value but nevertheless suggestive pointers. A man of sixty-five came into hospital with an acute coronary thrombosis. He admitted he had a heated quarrel with his girl friend who had refused to have sexual intercourse with him that night. A man of sixty who thought he had been cheated in a major business deal and was greatly enraged developed a stroke in this state of high emotion. A University professor who collapsed and died of a coronary thrombosis in the course of a retirement speech after a farewell banquet.

The link between emotion and vascular accidents should be pointed out to patients who are known to suffer from atherosclerosis with complications and they should be briefed to avoid situations of conflict and keep their calm to the best of their abilities. People are much more amenable to advice after their first cerebral or coronary thrombosis. Where discussion produces no results one could use mild tranquillizers such as Valium in small doses or β blockers which damp down sympathetic activity.

Hypertension is often associated with a restless, time-conscious personality. 'Hurry Disease' can be modified as described by Rosenman and Friedman in their book *Type A Behaviour and Your Heart.*[4]

Duodenal Ulcer

Patients with duodenal ulcers tend to have a high daytime secretion of acid and, as we have noted in our chapter on sleep, several peaks of acid secretion at night coinciding with REM periods. It is thought that there is an element of frustration, resentment and suppressed anger in the psychosocial situation. The work of Beaumont and Wolf and Wolff has shown the correlation between emotion and gastric appearance and secretion. This is not to say there are no other influences at work in the origin of the illness. For instance Blood Group O is commoner in patients with peptic ulcer, pointing to a hereditary element, and there is some evidence that diet, alcohol and tobacco all play a minor part.

Although some physicians tend to disregard dietary measures in treatment we feel that the least that should be done in this respect is for the patient to take regular, frequent and non-irritant meals each containing some starchy food. Gastric acid secretion can be partly inhibited by anticholinergic drugs like Probanthine and these may be taken before meals and at bedtime. Alkalis taken after meals help further to neutralize acid. A mild tranquillizer may be needed if there is interpersonal friction and tension.

It will be of great help to the patient if he can talk to his doctor about his problems and resentments. A good airing of his feelings will give him some insight into the psychological factors behind his illness, will lessen the pressure of his anger and permit him to see his problems in their correct perspective. The late Michael Balint, a physician interested in psychotherapy of psychosomatic disease, claimed in one of his case histories that he had cured a patient of his duodenal ulcer by the simple expedient of listening to him. He was probably right.

Alcohol is known to stimulate acid secretion and while there is pain it should be avoided altogether. Later a non-irritant dilute form could be drunk in moderation – possibly beer, or gin and tonic, or whisky and water and preferably with or after meals. Tobacco is also a gastric irritant and should be given up. But we have found little patient co-operation in this respect. Human nature is weak. Aspirin or aspirin-containing remedies are powerful irritants which may precipitate or aggravate an ulcer. Paracetamol is far safer. If need be, for example for rheumatic pain, one of the non-irritant forms of aspirin could be used.

Surgery should be rarely needed if medical treatment has been carefully planned and honestly carried out. It must be remembered that all surgery will interfere to some extent with normal structure and function. A portion of the stomach may be removed or the cholinergic fibres of the vagus can be cut. These operations are successful in the majority of patients who become pain free and comfortable but in a minority there will be complications such as fullness after meals, faintness, vomiting, ordinary or fatty diarrhoea and anaemias of one kind or another. There may be, in addition, a relapse of ulceration. All in all surgery cannot be lightly undertaken but only after a careful medical regime, which may include hospital admission, has been given a full chance.

The treatment of duodenal ulcer has been revolutionized in recent years by the introduction of Tagamet (cimetidine) which blocks H_2 receptors in the stomach lining thus preventing the secretion of Histamine and this lowers acid secretion to a greater extent than anticholinergic tablets. (It appears that in the production of gastric acid one of the first stimulants is acetylcholine, while histamine is the second.) This new form of treatment is so effective that the call for surgery has been greatly reduced. However, as the drug is extremely expensive it cannot be dispensed indiscriminately but only after X-ray proof of the existence of an ulcer.

Ulcerative Colitis

As with so many of the stress-linked diseases, the exact origin is unknown. There are almost certainly hereditary factors, witness the link with ankylosing spondylitis. Autoimmunity plays a part and some fifty per cent of patients will be found to have antibodies to their own colonic lining or to milk protein. An infective element is likely but specific organisms have not been pin-pointed. It used to be thought that mothers of affected patients had a specific personality, being excessively domineering and possessive and that, in consequence, the patients themselves became excessively attached, dependent and obsessional. There is no good evidence that this is so but only that emotional stress of many different varieties will precipitate or aggravate a disease to which the individual is, in any case, prone.

The illness is characterized by ulceration of portions of the large gut or even its entire length and, more rarely, it may also involve the terminal end of the small gut. This pathological picture is usually associated with diarrhoea, bleeding and pain together with symptoms of general ill-health and possibly fever.

In view of the possible role of infection in the disease it is not surprising that a sulphonamide combined with salicylic acid (salazopyrin) is effective especially in the milder cases. As with so many stress disorders cortico-steroids seem to be very useful. They can be given locally in the form of suppositories or retention enemas and this is the preferred way, or they can be given orally in the more severe cases, but obviously long continued treatment with steroids would give rise to harmful side-effects. Measures are taken to control diarrhoea, and these might include codeine phosphate and some bulk producing agent such as isogel. In keeping with the findings of abnormal autoimmune processes in the disease the immunosuppressive drugs, such as Imuran are sometimes helpful.

Interestingly enough cromoglycate (Intal) which is so useful in asthma, has now been found to be of value in some cases of ulcerative colitis, thus confirming the suspicion that there is an allergic element at play in this condition.

Psychotherapy is likely to be helpful in most cases, the intensity being adjusted to the need. Sensibly regulated rest and the sheltering or removal of the patient from traumatic relationships and social obligations are also required to raise the central resistance.

Surgery may become necessary as a result of some emergency or it may be invoked, on a carefully planned basis, if medical treatment is seen to be failing, or to forestall a possible complication. We should expect a gradual lessening of surgical procedures as our understanding of the disease increases and as we tackle its early stages more energetically, especially with adequate psychotherapy and rest.

Eczema

This is an inherited condition and can be one of the manifestations of the allergic triad Asthma, Hay Fever and Eczema. The onset, in babies, may be between the third and sixth month with redness, scaling, weeping, crusting and thickening of the skin in the face, neck, trunk and limbs. Immunoglobulin levels in the blood are raised, confirming the allergic nature of the disease but skin tests, which are often positive to a large range of foods, are not helpful as they are seldom a true reflection of the cause of the disease.

One wonders how emotional stress could possibly play a part at so early an age, but it probably does. Infants can be frustrated in many ways – by anxious, unstable, unpredictable mothers, by unsatisfactory feeding methods, by disturbance from siblings and by changes in the physical environment. When eczema makes its appearance it induces itching, scratching and loss of sleep and a vicious circle is set up of stress leading to eczema and eczema maintaining the state of stress, which results in the disease becoming self-perpetuating. If infantile eczema is not controlled, then, as the infant grows into a child, its character changes, and it becomes localized mainly to the flexures, that is the front of the elbows and the backs of the knees. The condition is usually self-limiting after a period of some months but it may become chronic. Adults may suffer from eczema, but the rash is more often in the nature of a contact dermatitis.

Hydrocortisone cream is applied to the area if it is weeping and ointment if it is dry. If there is a superimposed infection then an antibiotic such as neomycin or aureomycin may be added to the steroid preparation. The stronger, fluorinated cortico-steroids are avoided, as they can depress the function of the adrenal cortex and as they may cause, in addition, thinning of the skin. Antihistamine sedatives decrease itching and are helpful in encouraging sleep.

Psychotherapy is directed at the parents. A calm, stable handling of the infant is needed and interpersonal relationships between members of the family may need some adjustment. Parents' fears as to the outlook in eczema should be discussed and allayed. The fact is that with modern treatment eczema is not nearly the formidable disease it once was.

Psoriasis

Plaques of thickened skin with a silvery flaking of the superficial layers, sometimes coalescing, and being most prominent over knees and elbows characterize this skin disease which is a nuisance not so much by reason of pain, itching or general ill-health but simply because it is cosmetically unwelcome. Here again there is a hereditary basis. Psychological stress is often a precipitating factor while local trauma or pressure may determine where the lesions are most prolific. Fatigue may likewise encourage psoriasis.

Locally applied cortico-steroid ointments are moderately effective and their action can be enhanced by occlusive polythene dressings. But one has to bear in mind the danger of long continued treatment. So other means are frequently used or treatments are given in rotation. Coal tar applications are not so spectacular, but safer, and colourless and odourless preparations are available. A coal tar solution can be added to the daily bath.

Recent research has shown that ultraviolet light can be very effective in the treatment of Psoriasis if a chemical called Psoralen is given first. Another treatment which promises to be very useful has been developed in China.[5] The second messenger, one of the high energy phosphates, already referred to in the chapter on chronic fatigue, when given by injection as Dibutyryl AMP, has had considerable success in severe forms of Psoriasis. This treatment is not yet available in this country.

Non-specific stress situations should be investigated and the pressures on the patient be reduced. A good holiday has often cleared psoriasis away.

Dermatitis

Dermatitis means an inflammatory reaction in the skin, not usually bacterial but allergic in nature. Sensitive individuals may develop a dermatitis after only a short period of contact with the offending substance while the less sensitive take longer or remain unaffected. The range of chemicals which can bring about a dermatitis is vast. In the home it may be detergents, articles of clothing, dyes used in leather, chrome or nickel in metal objects. In the garden primula leaves, bulbs, insecticides. In industry a range of chemicals too numerous to mention. The exposed skin becomes red, swollen, weeping, crusted and possibly infected. Its distribution will often give a clue as to the nature of the responsible agent. Fatigue and mental stress are common precursors of the condition.

It is wise to remove the offending substance from the patient or the patient from the offending environment. Which reminds one of Oscar Wilde's remark on his deathbed. He was looking at some ugly wallpaper which he disliked. 'Either it or I will have to go!' Cortico-steroid creams or ointments with or without antibiotics are of value. It is just as well to help with any stress or fatigue situation. Tranquillizers or antidepressants might be needed for a time.

Urticaria

Urticaria is another allergic skin condition which is popularly referred to as nettle rash. There is a pink wheal of various sizes, often irregular in shape, affecting any part of the body, but especially areas which are scratched. A more severe variant affecting the orbits, and sometimes the tongue, is called Augioneurotic oedema. The wheals will persist for hours or days and new crops come up in different areas usually spontaneously, dying out over a period of weeks. The history and skin tests may incriminate strawberries, shell fish, pork or some other food but often no causal antigen is found. In this respect it must be remembered that there is a host of chemical preservatives and additives in canned and prepacked foods, making it a virtual impossibility to test for allergy to this vast range of substances. The onset, in allergic individuals, is often determined by a combination of stress, fatigue and the ingestion of the particular food to which the individual is sensitive.

Antihistamines are the main plank in treatment and should be given in adequate doses, taking care to warn the patient of possible soporific side effects. Soothing applications such as calamine lotion are applied locally. Offending foodstuffs, if known, are avoided wherever possible. Finally help is given with psychological problems and reasonable rest encouraged.

Conclusion

*

STRESS NEED NOT BE blindly avoided, for some measure of conflict, anxiety and stress is a natural and necessary ingredient of our daily lives and may indeed spur us on to greater effort and creativity; and yet we need to know the limit of tolerance to it and this will vary from individual to individual, for an overload will lead, as we have seen, to extreme physiological responses and, in some cases, to pathological changes and disease.

The view that some illnesses are almost wholly due to specific stresses, acting upon people with specific personality defects is no longer tenable and is being replaced by a broader concept – that some degree of stress plays a part in almost all disease, while being most prominent in the so-called 'psychosomatic' diseases. But even here it is recognized that heredity and specific conditioning factors determine the nature of the illness which may develop.

The Cluster theory of disease represents a great advance and has confirmed the belief that stressful experience increases our susceptibility to disease. It does not, however, help to explain the mechanism by which stress leads to disease. As we have seen Selye's General Adaptation Syndrome is not entirely convincing nor have any other satisfactory hypotheses emerged. We have introduced a new hypothesis – the concept of chronic fatigue and its impact on health. We do not claim that chronic fatigue is responsible for all diseases of stress; far from it. When we fail to adapt we may overreact and come to suffer from diseases caused by the overactivity of some system, for example hypertension in the case of the cardiovascular system or duodenal ulcer in the case of the stomach. But equally we may become exhausted. We have not been in the habit of taking any notice of brain fatigue. It has always been assumed that sleep, even of poor quality and inadequate duration, will put it right. It seems to us more likely that as research in neurophysiology progresses we shall find that important groups of brain cells may become exhausted and underactive and that, in consequence there will be an impairment of function of sectors of the endocrine system. This applies particularly to the pituitary-adrenal axis, the lynch pin of our resistance to stress, whose diminished performance is a vital component of the syndrome of chronic fatigue. A study of patients suffering from this syndrome reveals certain physiological changes and minor physical abnormalities which combine to produce a characteristic profile and permits easier recognition of the condition. It is in this group that we find sufferers from the rheumatic and allergic complaints that cause so much misery and invalidism; and it is here that preventive action can be so rewarding.

If there is a message in this book it is that, in our search for health and happiness, we should be prepared to learn about ourselves in respect of both body and mind, structure and function, so that we may better control our destiny by organizing the external environment to be less stressful and the internal environment to be more robust and adaptive. A deeper knowledge will also bring greater self-reliance and respect for others, as we come to realize that we are all endowed with a wonderful body – mind mechanism and potential. Just as the artist can create a magnificent work if he understands his tools, his materials and his environment, so can we create fulfilled human beings if we come to understand the material from which we are made and the way in which we react to the outside world.

There are many other benefits which will accrue from a deeper understanding of conflict, emotion and stress. In industry we have, in the past, concentrated too much on technical and economic aspects of production, and these attitudes have led to worship of profit and output at the expense of biological fulfilment. The realization that the often intolerable conditions of work and the inherent and widespread conflicts in industry lead not only to decreased production but also to serious mental and physical ill-health may bring about a reappraisal of our present methods and a reorganization of industry to foster better interpersonal relationships and more realistic demands on workers by hand or brain in keeping with their biological potential and needs.

Over the centuries we have weak-mindedly and almost unconsciously slipped into too great a reliance on drugs so that real threats are now posed to our health by alcohol, tobacco, drugs of addiction and the vast array of tranquillizers and hypnotics. Mass production and our relative wealth have made all these things too accessible. It is in this field that a greater insight into the mechanism of sleep and the emotions will lead to natural means of coping with insomnia and anxiety and lessen our frightening dependence on drugs. Although mental illness has not been discussed in depth here there is little doubt that an understanding, and correct handling, of stress will go a long way in its prevention.

We are living in an age of unparalleled violence at all levels. Hooliganism, terrorism, revolution and war are our daily experience. It is to be hoped that one of the long term by-products of our increased understanding of the physiology of the emotions will be a lessening of individual fear, anger and aggression and, as an extension of this, decreased violence and conflict in all social groupings.

An understanding of our biological selves, of the means by which we can adapt to stressful events and of the limits of our capacity to do so, should not be confined to scientists but should be the prerogative of us all and should help us to achieve some measure of contentment and real health.

References

*

Chapter 1

1 Wolf, S. and Wolff, H. G., *Human Gastric Function. An Experimental Study of a Man and his Stomach*. 2nd Edition, O.U.P., New York, 1947.

2 Cannon, Walter B., *Bodily Changes in Pain, Hunger, Fear and Rage*. D. Appleton and Co, New York and London, 1929.

3 Selye, Hans, *The Physiology and Pathology of Exposure to Stress*. Acta Inc, Montreal, 1950.

4 Funkenstein, D. H., King, S. H. and Drolette, Margaret E., *Mastery of Stress*. Harvard University Press, Cambridge, 1957.

5 Rahe, R. H., Mahan, J. L. Jr. and Arthur, R. J., 'Prediction of Near Future Health Change from Subjects' Preceding Life Changes', *Journal of Psychosomatic Research*, 14, 401-406, 1970.

6 Levi, Lennart (ed), *The Psychosocial Environment and Psychosomatic Diseases*. Vol. 1 : *Society, Stress and Disease*. O.U.P., London, 1971.

Chapter 2

1 Greisheimer, E. M. and Wiedeman, M. P., *Physiology and Anatomy*. J. B. Lippincott, Philadelphia, 1972.

Chapter 3

1 Cannon, Walter B., *op cit.*

Chapter 4

1 SELYE, Hans, *Nature*, 138, 32, 1936.
2 BAUER, W. and CLARK, W. S., *Recent Progress in Endocrine Research*. New York, 1953.
3 SELYE, Hans, in *Stress and Psychiatric Disorders*, edited by J. M. Tanner. Blackwell, Oxford, 1960.

Chapter 5

1 BASTIAANS, J. and GROEN, J., in *Modern Trends in Psychosomatic Medicine*, edited by Desmond O'Neill. Butterworth, London, 1955.
2 FRENCH, T. M. and ALEXANDER, F., 'Psychogenic Factors in Bronchial Asthma', in *Psychosomatic Medicine Monograph 3*. 1941.
3 FRENCH, T. M., ALEXANDER, F. and POLLOCK, G. H., *Psychosomatic Specificity*. University of Chicago Press, Chicago and London, 1968.
4 PINKERTON, P. and WEAVER, Corinna M., 'Childhood Asthma' in *Modern Trends in Psychosomatic Medicine, 2*, edited by O. W. Hill, Butterworth, London, 1970.
5 GARNETT, R. W., *Virginia Medical Monthly*, 82, 61, 1955.
6 GILLESPIE, R. D., *British Medical Journal*, I, 1285, 1936.
7 ELLMAN, P. and MITCHELL, S. D., 'The Psychological Aspects of Chronic Rheumatic Joint Disease', in *Reports on Chronic Rheumatic Diseases*, edited by W. Buckley. Macmillan, New York, 1936.
8 ALEXANDER, F., *Psychosomatic Medicine*. W. W. Norton, New York, 1956.
9 MOOS, R. H. and SOLOMON, G. F., 'Studies of Rheumatoid Arthritis Patients', in *Modern Trends in Psychosomatic Medicine, 2*. 1970.
10 O'CONNOR, J. F., 'A Comprehensive Approach to the Treatment of Ulcerative Colitis' in *Modern Trends in Psychosomatic Medicine, 2*. 1970.

Chapter 6

1 HOLMES, T. H. and RAHE, R. H., 'The Social Readjustment

Rating Scale' in *Journal of Psychosomatic Research*, 11, 213, 1967.

2 RAHE, R. H., MAHAN, J. L. Jr. and ARTHUR, R. J., 'Prediction of Near Future Health Change from Subjects' preceding Life Changes', in *Journal of Psychosomatic Research*, 14, 401, 1970.

3 RAHE, R. H., MCKEAN, J. D., and ARTHUR, R. J., 'A Longitudinal Study of Life Change and Illness Patterns', in *Journal of Psychosomatic Research*, 10, 355, 1967.

4 WYLER, A. R., MASUDA, M. and HOLMES, T. H., 'Magnitude of Life Events and Seriousness of Illness', in *Psychosomatic Medicine*, 33, 115, 1971.

5 HOLMES, T. S. and HOLMES, T. H., 'Short Term Intrusions into the Life Style Routine', in *Journal of Psychosomatic Research*, 14, 121, 1970.

Chapter 7

1 HEMINGWAY, A., *Nature*, 169, 728, 1952.

2 BARTLEY, S. H., *Fatigue, Mechanism and Management*. Charles C. Thomas, Illinois, 1965.

3 BROWNE, R. C., Fatigue, Fact or Fiction. *Symposium on Fatigue, The Ergonomics Research Society*, edited by Ffloyd and Welford, H. K. Lewis, 1953.

4 SPAULDING, W. B., 'The Clinical Analysis of Fatigue', in *Applied Therapeutics*, 6, 911, 1964.

5 GROOVER, M. E., 'An Unusual Syndrome Responding to Prolonged ACTH Therapy', in *Journal of the American Geriatrics Society*, 12, 350, 1964.

6 NÜSSBAUM, H. E., *Journal of the Medical Society of New Jersey*, 60, 499, 1963.

7 HELD, 'La Fatigue', in *Travaux du IIIe Congrès International de Medecine Psychosomatique*. Privat E., Toulouse, 1967.

Chapter 8

1 HENNEMAN, P. H., WANG, D. M. K., IRWIN, J. W. and BURRAGE, W. S., *Journal of the American Medical Association*, 158, 384, 1955.

2 COPEMAN, W. S. C., *Cortisone and ACTH*, page 39. London, 1953.
3 POTELIAKHOFF, A., 'Adrenocortical Activity and some Clinical Findings in Acute and Chronic Fatigue', in Journal of Psychosomatic Research, 25, 91, 1981.

Chapter 9

1 POTELIAKHOFF, A., *op. cit.*

Chapter 10

1 *Concepts of Sleep*. Roche, 1965.
2 *Sleep: Physiology and Pathology. A Symposium*, edited by Anthony Kales. Lippincott, Philadelphia, 1969.
3 ADAM, K., OSWALD, I., 'Sleep is for Tissue Restoration', in *Journal of the Royal College of Physicians of London*, 11 (no 4), 376, 1977.
4 TUNE, G. S., 'Sleep and Wakefulness in Normal Human Adults', *British Medical Journal*, 2, 269, 1968.
5 GERMAN, Allen G., and STAMPFER, H. G., Letter 'Hypothalmic Releasing Factor for Reactive Depression', *Lancet* 2, page 789, 1979.

Chapter 11

1 LAZARUS, R. S., AVERILL, J. R. and OPTON, E. M. in *Society, Stress and Disease, op cit*, page 190.
2 MORUZZI, G. and MAGOUN, H. W., 'Brain Stem Reticular Formation and Activation of the EEG', in *Electroencephalography and Clinical Neurophysiology*, I, 455, 1949.
3 SMYTHIES, J. R., *Brain Mechanisms and Behaviour*, Blackwell, Oxford, 1970.
4 PAPEZ, J. W., 'A Proposed Mechanism of Emotion', in *Archives of Neurology and Psychiatry*, 38, 725, 1937.
5 SMYTHIES, J. R., *op cit.*
6 HALL, G. H. and TURNER, D. M., 'Effects of Nicotine on the Release of Noradrenaline from the Hypothalamus', in *Biochemical Pharmacology*, 21, 1829, 1972.

7 SCHACHTER, S., 'Nesbitt's Paradox', in Dunn, W. L. (ed), *Smoking Behaviour: Motives and Incentives*. Winston, Washington DC, 1973.
8 FRANKENHAEUSER, M., in *Society, Stress and Disease, op cit*, page 22.
9 HEIMSTRA, N. W., BANCROFT, N. R. and DEKOCK, A. R., 'The Effects of Cigarette Withdrawal on Performance during Simulated Driving', *Annals of NY Academy of Sciences*, 142, 295, 1967.
10 LAUSCH, Erwin, *Manipulation*. Aidan Ellis, England, 1974.
11 FUNKENSTEIN, D. H., KING, S. H. and DROLETTE, M. E., *Mastery of Stress, op cit.*
12 ELMADJIAN, F. J., HOPE, J. and LAMSON, E. T., 'Excretion of Epinephrine and Norepinephrine in Various Emotional States', in *Journal of Clinical Endocrinology*, 17, 608, 1957.
13 FRANKENHAEUSER, M., *Society, Stress and Disease, op cit*, page 22.
14 BREGGEN, P. R., 'The Psychophysiology of Anxiety: with a Review of the Literature concerning Adrenaline', in *Journal of Nervous and Mental Diseases*, 139, 558, 1964.
15 JAMES, W., *Principles of Psychology*. Holt, New York, 1890.
16 CARRUTHERS, M. and MURRAY, A., *F/40: Fitness on 40 minutes per week*. Futura Books, London, 1976.
17 MYAGER, Valentina, 'Psychic Trauma and Cortical-Diencephalic Interrelationships', in *Society, Stress and Disease, op cit*, page 254.

Chapter 12

1 *Society, Stress and Disease, op cit.*
2 KAGAN, A. R. and LEVI, L., 'Health and Environment – Psychosocial Stimuli. A Review', in *Reports from the Laboratory of Clinical Stress Research*, no 27. Karolinska Institute, Stockholm, Dec., 1971.
3 CARLSON, L. A., LEVI, L. and ORO, L., in *Emotional Stress, Physiological and Psychological Reactions: Medical, Industrial and Military Implications*, (ed) Levi. Basel, 1967.
4 FROBERG, J., KARLSSON, C. G., LEVI, L., LIDBERG, L., and SEEMAN, K. 'Conditions of Work and their Influence on

Psychological and Endocrine Stress Reactions', in *Report no 8, Laboratory of Clinical Stress Research*, Archives of Environmental Health, 21, 789, 1969.
5 TAGGART, P., CARRUTHERS, M., and SOMERVILLE, W., 'Electrocardiogram, Plasma Catecholamines and Lipids and their Modification by Oxprenolol when Speaking before an Audience', *The Lancet*, 2, 341, 1973.
6 *Occupational Mortality*, Decennial Supplement, 1970–1972, England and Wales. Office of Population Censuses and Surveys, 1978.
7 *Rheumatism and Arthritis in Britain*. Office of Health Economics, 1973.
8 *The Common Illnesses of our Time. A Study of the Problems of Ischaemic Heart Disease*. Office of Health Economics, 1966.
9 SHIROM, A., and others, *Society, Science and Medicine*, 7, 875, 1973.
10 BAXTER, P. J. and others, *British Journal of Industrial Medicine*, 33, 1, 1976.
11 RUSSEK, H. I. and ZOHMAN, B. L., *Changing Concepts in Cardiovascular Disease*. Williams and Wilkins, Baltimore, 1972.
12 FRIEDMAN, M. and ROSENMAN, R. H., *Type A Behaviour and Your Heart*. Knopf, New York, 1974.
13 REEDER, L. G. and others. *Society, Science and Medicine*, 7, 573, 1973.
14 COBB, S. and ROSE, R. M., 'Hypertension, Peptic Ulcer and Diabetis in Air Traffic Controllers', in *Journal of the American Medical Association*, 224, 489, 1973.
15 MELTON, C. E. and others, *Stress in Air Traffic Controllers*. FAA Office of Aviation Medicine Report, no FAA, A17–75–7, 1975.
16 OSTBERG, O., 'Interindividual Differences in Circadian Fatigue Patterns of Shiftworkers', in *British Journal of Industrial Medicine*, 30, 341, 1973.
17 THEORELL, T. and AKERSTEDT, T., *Acta Medica Scandinavia*, 200, 47, 1976.
18 BROWNE, R. C., *Health in Industry*. Edward Arnold, London, 1961.
19 CARRUTHERS, M. and MURRAY, A., *F/40: Fitness in 40 minutes per week, op cit*.

20 BROOK, A., 'Mental Stress at Work' in *The Practitioner*, 210, 500, 1973.
21 SHIMMIN, Sylvia, 'People and Work. Some contemporary Issues', in *British Journal of Industrial Medicine*, 32, 93, 1975.

Chapter 13

1 *The Encyclopedia of Psychiatry for General Practitioners*, Roche, 1972.
2 JERSILD, A. T., *Child Psychology.* Staples Press, London, 1969.
3 MILLER, N. E., 'Psychosomatic Effects of Specific Types of Training', in *Annals of New York Academy of Science*, 159, article 3, 1025, 1969.
4 LUCE, G. G., *Body Time.* Palladin, St Albans, 1973.
5 DUFFY, E., 'The Concept of Energy Mobilisation', in *Psychological Review*, 58, 30, 1951.
6 LADER, M. H., 'The Responses of Normal Subjects and Psychiatric Patients to Repetitive Stimulation', in *Society, Stress and Disease, op cit.*

Chapter 14

1 ROBERTS, C. A., 'Primary Prevention of Psychiatric Disorders' in *Society, Stress and Disease, op cit*, page 369.
2 SARGANT, W., *The Mind Possessed.* Heinemann, London, 1973.

Chapter 15

1 AITKEN, R. C. B., ROSENTHAL, S. V., and ZEALLY, A. K., 'The Cattell 16PF Personality Profile of Asthmatics', in *Journal of Psychological Research*, 17, 9, 1973.

Chapter 16

1 HENRY, J. P., MEEHAN, F. P. and STEPHENS, P. M., 'The Use of Psychosocial Stimuli to Induce Prolonged Systolic

Hypertension in Mice', in *Psychosomatic Medicine*, 29, 408, 1967.

2 PATEL, C., NORTH, W. R. S., 'Randomised Controlled Trial of Yoga and Bio-Feedback in Management of Hypertension', in *The Lancet*, 2, 93, 1975.

3 CARRUTHERS, M. and MURRAY, A., *F/40: Fitness in 40 minutes per week*, *op cit*.

4 FRIEDMAN, M. and ROSENMAN, R. H., *Type A Behaviour and Your Heart*, *op cit*.

5 Department of Dermatology, 'Cyclic AMP and Dibutyryl AMP in Treatment of Psoriasis' in *Chinese Medicine*, 2, 141, 1976.

Index

*